Acute Renal Failure

Acute Renal Failure

Edited by
C.T. Flynn

Springer-Science+Business Media, B.V.

Originally published by MTP in 1974
Softcover reprint of the hardcover 1st edition 1974

ISBN 978-94-010-9081-0 ISBN 978-94-010-9079-7 (eBook)
DOI 10.1007/978-94-010-9079-7

Blackburn Times Ltd
Blackburn, Lancashire

CONTENTS

ACKNOWLEDGEMENTS

I would like to thank the Director General of Medical Services (RAF) for his permission to arrange the Symposium, and to the Commandant, RAF Halton, and his staff, for generous help and the use of the Station's facilities.
I am grateful to the many people who helped and advised me and in particular to my secretary, Lynda Rance, whose memory for details and capacity for hard work exceeded mine, and to Flying Officer John Simms, Medical Administrator Extraordinary, who translated my vague impressions of what might be needed into a smooth faultless organisation.
Finally, I would like to record my appreciation for the help given by Baxter Travenol for supporting the Symposium.

C.T. FLYNN

LIST OF SPEAKERS AND THEIR ADDRESSES

Dr A M Joekes, FRCP
Consultant Physician,
St Philip's Hospital,
Sheffield Street,
LONDON, W.C.2

Professor D N S Kerr, FRCP
Department of Medicine,
Wellcome Research Laboratories,
Royal Victoria Infirmary,
NEWCASTLE UPON TYNE NE1 4LP

Dr T Sherwood, MRCP, FFR, DMRD
Senior Lecturer in Radiology,
Institute of Urology,
172 Shaftesbury Avenue,
LONDON, WC2H 8JE

Dr Claus Brun,
Central Clinical Laboratory,
Kommunehospitalet,
5, Ø Farimugsgade,
COPENHAGEN K,
Denmark

Professor W F O'Dwyer, MD, FRCPI
Physician in Charge of Renal Department and
Artificial Kidney Unit,
Jervis Street Hospital,
DUBLIN, 1

Dr D K Peters, MRCP
Lecturer in Medicine and Immunology,
Consultant Physician,
Department of Medicine,
Royal Postgraduate Medical School,
Hammersmith Hospital,
LONDON, W12

Dr D B Evans, MRCP
Consultant Physician,
Renal Transplant Unit,
New Addenbrooke's Hospital,
Haverhill Road,
CAMBRIDGE

Dr R M Lindsay, MRCP
Associate Director,
Renal Unit,
Victoria Hospital,
London,
ONTARIO,
Canada

Dr C T Flynn, MBE, MRCP
Consultant in Medicine,
Renal Unit,
Princess Mary's RAF Hospital,
Halton,
AYLESBURY,
Bucks

EDITORIAL

Nowadays a doctor with adequate means of support could spend most of his time attending Medical Meetings or Symposia. Some justification is therefore required for this Symposium on Acute Renal Failure, and for publishing it.

In this country it is ten years since the last major symposium devoted entirely to acute renal failure was held at the Royal Free Hospital, London. At that time the participants were enthusiasts largely convinced of the value of dialytic therapy in renal failure. It was also the time when the extension of dialysis to the long term treatment of patients with chronic renal failure was an exciting prospect. That symposium was also a crucial event leading to the formation of the European Dialysis and Transplant Association. In the next ten years the complex related problems of chronic haemodialysis and renal transplantation have occupied the interests and energies of most nephrologists and the advances made have been an outstanding feature in the astonishing progress in nephrology as a whole. During this time acute renal failure receded from being a dominant topic of interest, even though many advances in our understanding of its pathogenesis, investigations and treatment have been made. The introduction of peritoneal dialysis has allowed many patients to be treated without transfer to a renal unit. The advantages of this are obvious and were welcomed by many units already overburdened with chronic renal failure patients. Against these advantages must be set that the incidence, mortality and changing pattern of acute renal failure have become conjecture rather than fact, and the possibility that some patients are deprived of the expertise that a modern renal unit can offer. A simple questionnaire designed to gather some information on the incidence and current attitudes to the treatment of acute renal failure was sent to 35 renal units, and is presented in the Appendix. No less than 34 replies were received which, in this age of questionnaires, speaks for itself. Only 26 were complete, or available in time, to be presented at the symposium and, because several people have wished to quote these figures, they are given in the chapter on the Treatment of Acute Renal Failure.

Dr A.M. Joekes, the pioneer of haemodialysis in this country, gives an account of acute renal failure in the past 25 years. This is followed by chapters on pathogenesis, radiology and renal biopsy each of which sheds light of our understanding on acute renal failure. The next three chapters are selected aspects of acute renal failure which illustrate its diversity, namely in pregnancy, glomerulonephritis and renal transplantation. The final chapters are concerned with the factors in prognosis and selected aspects of treatment.

The Symposium was attended by doctors from almost every renal unit in the U.K. and Ireland. It augurs well for the future that acute renal failure continues to excite their interest. I would like to offer my thanks to the contributors whose enthusiasm made the symposium possible and to the participants in the lively discussions that followed all their papers.

C.T. FLYNN

OPENING ADDRESS – By Air Marshal Sir Ernest Sidey, KBE QHP MD ChB MFCM

It gives me great pleasure to welcome you to this Symposium on Acute Renal Failure. It is I believe about ten years since a gathering of this nature took place to discuss this condition and the fact that this meeting today has aroused such widespread interest is evidenced by the number here this morning; round about the 200 mark. The fact that so many eminent civilian clinicians have found it worthwhile, not only to come here this morning but also to give papers, must indeed by very gratifying to the organisers and the sponsors and in this respect I would pay tribute to Wing Commander Flynn who has borne the brunt of the organising and to Baxters of Travenol Laboratories to whom we are indeed grateful for their very generous financial support.

I am particularly pleased that it has been decided to hold this meeting at Halton, if for no other reason than that on the advice of Air Vice Marshal Sir Aubrey Rumball and Dr. Joekes it was decided in 1957 to establish the first Kolff twin-coil artificial kidney unit in the U.K. at Princess Mary's R.A.F. Hospital, Halton. The officer in charge of that unit at that time in 1957 was Group Captain R.C. Jackson, now Air Vice Marshal Sir Ralph Jackson, Senior Consultant to the Royal Air Force. The contribution that he has made in the field that we are discussing this morning, the use of the artificial kidney, is known and justifiably recognised not only in this country but overseas as well. It is also appropriate that our first speaker this morning should be Dr Joekes who is still the Civil Consultant in Renal Disorders to the Royal Air Force.

In June 1957 the first patient was treated at Halton Hospital, a patients suffering from renal failure due to accidental trauma, and a new era really began in the treatment of this condition. The next development was the mobile artificial kidney unit and this has been used extensively in Service and civilian hospitals in the United Kingdom, and overseas in our hospitals in Cyprus, Singapore, Malta and Germany.

In 1957 at the same time as the Royal Air Force was establishing this unit at Halton, Mr. Ralph Shackman was establishing a rotating-drum artificial kidney at the Royal Postgraduate Hospital, Hammersmith and Dr. Frank Parsons was also operating a similar kidney unit at Leeds Royal Infirmary. It is most appropriate that Mr. Shackman, an ex-Wing Commander in the Royal Air Force Medical Branch is with us this morning and I welcome him back to the fold.

I believe that you will find this Symposium today of great value and without further ado I would like to hand you over now to your Chairman for this morning's session, Sir Ralph Jackson.

Chapter 1

ACUTE REVERSIBLE RENAL FAILURE; THE LAST 25 YEARS

As good may come out of evil so World Wars 1 and 2 were responsible for the rediscovery of acute renal failure following severe injury. In World War 1 the first attempts at large scale blood transfusion were not infrequently followed by renal damage accepted as being due to intravascular haemolysis. Kidney damage was also recognised at this time as complicating trauma, in particular that occurring in burial in bombed buildings.

World War 2 led to the recognition of 'crush syndrome', interpreted as the result of severe crushing or other muscle injury. In the interim between the wars acute traumatic kidney damage had been ignored. Initially, the main interest during the second World War was in establishing the histology of the crush kidney lesion[1,2] and in attempting animal experimental work which might clarify the aetiological factors.

The approach to treatment was mainly nihilistic, as it had been to any other form of uraemia in the past, and it was confidently expected that a patient with the crush syndrome would die within two weeks of the onset of the kidney failure.

In Holland, Borst[3] emphasised the importance of restricted protein intake in the management of renal failure, without particular reference to acute kidney damage. In the small provincial town of Kampen, Kolff recognised that, with commercially available cellophane tubing as a cheap and reliable dialysing membrane and with the production of heparin by Jorpes in Sweden as a safe anticoagulant, it should be possible to overcome the previous problems of clinical haemodialysis with an artificial kidney[4]. The gift by Kolff of one of his six original artificial kidneys to Hammersmith Hospital, with the dietetic approach by Borst as a further stimulus, was the starting point for the study and treatment of acute reversible renal failure in that centre. Although as early as 1947 we had a small number of patients who had been treated with haemodialysis during an episode of acute renal failure and recovered[5], the technical problems with the original Kolff artificial kidney were considerable, with the most important being the very large potential extracorporeal blood volume.

Observing patients in acute renal failure the immediate cause of the fatal outcome appeared in almost all cases to be left heart failure. The single most important cause seemed to be water overload, and it was striking that patients who had been 'actively' treated in hospital were usually in a far worse clinical condition than those who came straight from their home or had only briefly been in another hospital. It was not until estimation of plasma potassium concentration by flame photometer was possible and direct writing electrocardiography became available that the importance of hyperkalaemia was clearly established as an important immediate cause of death due to cardiac arrest. Apart from the retention of the excess intake of water, the inevitable accumulation of protein metabolites led to the progressive acidosis and haemostatic disturbances of severe renal failure. We adopted the simple therapeutic approach of not putting into the patient that which would not come out in the urine. From this developed the simplified artificial diet of an emulsion of arachis oil in glucose solution, with one litre of this mixture given per 24 hours and containing 2400 calories with no sodium, potassium or proteins, but reducing tissue catabolism to a minimum. Out of a series of 11 patients with acute renal failure treated by this simple conservative regime seven survived[6], and a certain euphoria was engendered which led to the belief that acute reversible oliguric renal failure had only to be treated by such a strict conservative management and recovery was to be expected. All too soon the continued high fatality rate of acute reversible renal failure made it clear that while the conservative management must be the essential basis of treatment, other measures would be necessary if more successful results were to be achieved.

Mathé and Crosnier made a very important contribution to the conservative management of patients by emphasising the importance of the water of metabolism which amounted to 400–500 ml/24 hours in an adult[7]. In our own regime we had based the water requirements on the insensible water loss at 1 litre/24 hours with an additional volume of water equal to the urine, vomit or diarrhoea lost in the preceeding 24 hours. This ignored the water of metabolism and on such a regime a patient would receive an excess of about 5 litres of water in a ten-day period.

With the continued high death rate in acute renal failure in patients following trauma, major surgery, burns or associated with or complicated by sepsis, despite careful conservative management, various methods of eliminating waste products were increasingly used. With the scarcity of artificial kidney machines and the considerable complications of their use, haemodialysis was virtually discontinued for a number of years. Peritoneal dialysis or gastroenterostinal lavage were used in many centres but the results were disappointing in the group of patients with the high catabolism. From the mid-1950s several artifical kidneys with fixed, or relatively fixed, extracorporeal blood volume were developed. In Copenhagen, Brun using a multi-layer Skeggs–Leonards type of flat kidney with a very high clearance rate, was probably the first to have a major improvement of the results in patients with a high catabolic rate. In 1957 the newly developed twin-coil kidney by Kolff was introduced at Halton in their very successful acute renal failure unit which has contributed so much in this country. Teschan, in the United States, convincingly demonstrated the value of early and repeated, often daily, haemodialysis in patients with renal failure following trauma[8]. There is little doubt that most specialised units dealing with the acute renal failure patients with high catabolic rates now use early elective haemodialysis.

The relatively disappointing overall results of acute reversible renal failure as seen in specialised units is a reflection of the reluctance of general physicians or surgeons to refer the patients with acute reversible renal failure to specialised centres. There is little doubt that because of this reluctance many potentially recoverable patients are not surviving. Only when the patient is obviously critically ill or has major complications associated with the renal failure are the patients usually referred to a specialised unit.

Trueta *et al.*[9] were the first to attempt an explanation of the causative factors of acute renal failure following trauma or shock by a study of the renal circulation. By the use of *in vivo* angiograms of kidneys after death, they were able for the first time to demonstrate two main blood-flow territories in the kidney. The one through the cortex was fast and the other through the medulla was much slower. Following renal or sciatic nerve stimulation the cortical blood flow was grossly reduced whereas the medullary flow was unchanged. These observations led to the general misinterpretation of the presence of an intrarenal 'shunt'. Nevertheless, they were an outstanding technical achievement and their basic validity has been fully established.

Bull, Joekes and Lowe[10] studied renal function in 33 patients with oliguric renal failure with a wide spectrum of different aetiological causes including trauma and poisoning. Glomerular filtration and effective renal blood flow measured by *para*-aminohippurate (PAH) were both found to be grossly reduced during the oliguric phase. With the use of renal vein catheterization it was possible to measure the extraction ratio of PAH across the kidney and obtain a measurement of renal blood flow by the direct Flick method. By this method the renal blood flow was also found to be grossly reduced to something of the order of 5% during the oliguric phase. Renal arteriovenous oxygen differences were either the same or greater than normal and this was accepted as evidence against the presence of any significant intrarenal shunt.

These authors used 'acute tubular necrosis' as a descriptive diagnostic term and divided the clinical course of this potentially reversible lesion into four phases: (i) onset; (ii) oliguric; (iii) early diuretic; and (iv) late diuretic.

During phases (ii) and (iii) the renal tubules were unable to concentrate urea and creatinine, to extract PAH, to reabsorb glucose at a normal rate and, of particular clinical importance, in phase (iii) to conserve sodium, potassium or chloride.

Sirota[11] studied four patients with acute renal failure following poisoning with mercury and obtained essentially the same results as regards renal haemodynamics and function.

In Denmark, Brun and Munck and their colleagues[12] adapted the techniques for measuring cerebral flow with radioactive krypton to the estimation of renal blood flow in patients with 'acute anuric renal failure'. As in the findings by Suc, who used the nitrous oxide method, the renal blood flow measured in six cases[13] gave mean values of 159 ml/100 g min in the oliguric phase and 114 ml/100 g min in the diuretic phase, compared with a normal of 420 ml/100 g min. The blood flow in these patients with acute renal failure was in the region of 30% of normal as opposed to the 5% according to the findings of Bull, Joekes and Lowe.

This higher value for the blood flow was also found in similar patients by Shaldon using indocyanin green[14]. Following a bolus of the dye into a renal artery the disappearance rate from the renal vein blood was interpreted as a measure of the renal blood flow assuming the kidney to be a perfect mixing chamber. Subsequently the more sophisticated mathematical handling of the concentration – time curve obtained by external scintillation monitoring following an intrarenal bolus of krypton-85 or xenon-133 – established that the reduction in renal blood flow is mainly in the cortical area with a relatively intact medullary blood flow[15,16].

It is interesting to speculate why the results by the direct Fick method should have given such falsely low results. It was suggested by Brun *et al.*[12] that the very low extraction ratios found could account for the inaccuracy of the method. However, the values were surprisingly uniform in those patients studied by Bull *et al.* and did not show the random scatter that would be expected from technical inaccuracy, and some other explanation seemed likely. In the direct Fick method it is assumed that the removal of PAH from the blood by the kidneys is into a single compartment, namely the urine. With radioactive renography, using the PAH analogue *o*-iodohippurate, serial observations in oliguric or *totally anuric* patients may show progressive shortening of the half-time of the tissue disappearance curve as well as evidence of increasing renal uptake over several days either while the patient remains anuric or while there is no increase in renal function measured by creatinine clearance[17]. This renographic investigation has proved to be of invaluable prognostic significance in patients with acute renal failure and particularly in the immediate post-operative period in homo-transplanted kidneys. The explanation must be that the kidney tubules retain or regain the ability to concentrate *o*-iodohippurate either in the epithelial cells or into a tubular filtrate which is subsequently reabsorbed.

In attempting to use the direct Fick principle in patients with oliguric renal failure there is a two compartmental system one of which, that in the kidney, is not estimated. Theoretically the blood flow should, therefore, be derived from $(UV + K)/(A - V)$, where K = kidney content and (A - V) = extraction ratio of PAH. Obviously, the Fick principle cannot be used to measure blood flow in oliguric renal failure and this explains the discrepancy between this method and more direct techniques.

It must be emphasised that not all patients with acute tubular necrosis or dysfunction are oliguric. Acute renal failure following head injuries is frequently followed by a renal failure with maintained urine flow. The management of such patients is similar to that of patients in the early diuretic phase with careful replacement of measured water and electrolyte losses until the late diuretic phase occurs when the tubules regain the ability to maintain homeostasis and increase U/P of urea and creatinine.

Although the early diuretic phase is more commonly associated with an irrational loss of sodium and to a less extent of potassium, observations at Halton[18] demonstrated that a severe sodium conservation following trauma may be seen both in the oliguric and early diuretic phases, which is not affected by iatrogenic hypernatraemia. The replacement of sodium and potassium during the early diuretic phase should, therefore, be on the basis of measurement of urinary losses and cannot safely be estimated.

No attempt will be made to review the enormous amount of experimental work which has be devoted to elucidating the mechanism of the onset of acute renal failure. To the clinician the interest must lie in therapeutic procedures which prevent or reverse the intrarenal haemodynamic changes which result in established acute tubular dysfunction. The elegant radiological observations of the renal blood flow following bleeding in dogs by Lavender and Sherwood[19] re-emphasised the importance of correcting hypovolaemia. Equally important is the correction of water and electrolyte depletion. Only when these prerenal factors have been corrected should other attempts at instituting a diuresis be used.

There have been two main lines of approach to reversing the intrarenal factors causing the renal failure. The most frequently used and certainly with the best documented evidence is the induction of an osmotic diuresis by rapid intravenous administration of 20–25% mannitol, usually in a volume of 200 ml[20]. There can be few people handling patients with acute reversible renal failure who have not seen an immediate and dramatic response with such an infusion. A possible explanation is that, even in the presence of anuria, some glomerular filtration persists but that little or none of the filtered sodium passes beyond the proximal tubule and that a feedback mechanism at the juxta-glomerular apparatus leads to the persistence of the haemodynamic changes, with cortical shut-down possibly through the renin–angiotensin mechanism. Osmotic diuresis induced by mannitol could carry sodium to the juxta-glomerular apparatus and so inhibit the feedback mechanism. It is certainly striking that almost in every case where a dramatic diuresis is achieved with mannitol the diuresis persists and there is a relatively rapid return of renal concentrating ability.

The diuretic frusemide has been claimed to reverse the early stages of acute tubular dysfunction, but it has not been possible to confirm this from our own observations. In a small number of our patients in acute oliguria with renal dysfunction following open-heart surgery, who have failed to respond to mannitol or frusemide, a diuresis has followed a single intravenous dose of ethacrynic acid (50 mg).

The other approach to reversing or possibly preventing acute renal dysfunction has aimed at altering intrarenal vascular resistance. Renal denervation by spinal block has been claimed to prevent the onset of renal failure but there is little in the way of concrete documentation. More recently, there is good evidence that an adrenergic alpha-blocking agent, phenoxybenzamine, can reverse the early stage of experimental oliguric renal failure[21]. It has been used extensively in the pre-agonal phase in patients in whom it is intended to utilise cadaver donor kidneys. There is also some evidence that acetylcholine may prevent or possibly reverse the haemodynamic changes in experimental acute renal dysfunction.

At one time the use of dextran was advocated in open-heart surgery in order to prevent the alterations in intrarenal haemodynamics. In an unpublished series[22] of observations on eight patients receiving Rheomacrodex during cardiac surgery, one of the patients developed a classical acute tubular dysfunction with eventual recovery. In these observations it became clear that the use of Rheomacrodex resulted in a sodium antidiuresis, probably because of plasma dilution with hyponatraemia.

Finally, only the early recognition soon after the onset phase of acute renal dysfunction by physicians and surgeons will allow correction of prerenal factors and an attempt to induce a diuresis with an osmotic load, diuretics or intrarenal vascular dilatation to be attempted in time. In our experience it is rarely possible to reverse the early dysfunction phase after 36 hours and never after 48 hours from the onset. It cannot too often be restated that the recognition of the early stages of acute renal dysfunction *can* only be made from the characteristics of the urine, with the concentrations of urea or creatinine as the fundamentally important measurement.

References

1. Dunn, J.S., Gillespie, M. and Niven, J.S.F. (1941). *Lancet,* **2,** 549
2. Bywaters, E.G.L. and Dible, J.H. (1942). *J. Path. Bart.,* **54,** 111
3. Borst, J.G.G. (1948). *Lancet,* **1,** 824
4. Kolff, W.J. (1944). *Acta Med. Scand.,* **117,** 121
5. Bywaters, E.G.L. and Joekes, A.M. (1948). *Proc. Roy. Soc. Med.,* **41,** 420
6. Bull, G.M., Joekes, A.M. and Lowe, K.G. (1949). *Lancet,* **2,** 229
7. Mathe, G. and Crosnier, J. (1950). *J. d'Urol.,* **56,** 760
8. Teschan, P.E., O'Brian, T.F. and Baxter, C.R. (1960). *U.S. Armed Forces. Med. J.* , **11,** 991
9. Trueta, J., Barclay, A.E., Daniel, P.M., Franklin, K.J. and Prichard, M.M.L. (1947). *Studies of the Renal Circulation* (Springfield: Charles C Thomas)
10. Bull, G.M., Joekes, A.M. and Lowe, K.G. (1950). *Clin. Sci.,* **9,** 379
11. Sirota, J.H. (1949). *J. Clin. Invest.,* **28,** 1412
12. Brun, C., Crone, C., Davidsen, H.G., Fabricus, J., Tybjaerg Hansen, A., Lassen, N.A. and Munck, O. (1955). *Proc. Soc. Exp. Biol.,* **89** 687
13. Munck, O. (1955). *Renal Circulation in Acute Renal Failure.* (Oxford: Blackwell Scientific Publications).
14. Shaldon, S., Walker, J.G., Lawson, J.R., Ryder, J., and Sylvan, H. (1963). *Proc. Soc. Exp. Biol.,* **112,** 932
15. Carriere, S., Thorburn, G.D., O'Morchoe, C.C.C. and Barger, A.C. (1966). *Circulation Res.,* **19,** 167
16. Hollenberg, N.K., Epstein, M., Rosen, S.M., Basch, R.I., Oken, D.E. and Merrill, J.P. (1968). *Medicine, Balt.,* **47,** 455
17. Constable, A.R., Hyne, B.E. and Joekes, A.M. Unpublished data
18. Elder, J. Unpublished data
19. Lavender, J.P. and Sherwood, T. (1972). *Brit. Med. Bull.,* **28,** 241
20. Barry, K.G. and Malloy, J.P. (1962). *J. Amer. Med. Assn.,* **179,** 510
21. Grandchamp, A., Veyrat, R., Strebel, H. and Truniger, B. (1972). *Radionuclides in Nephrology,* (New York, and London: Grune and Stratton).
22. Ghose, R.R. and Joekes, A.M. Unpublished observations.

Chapter 2

THE PATHOGENESIS OF ACUTE RENAL FAILURE

D.N.S. Kerr and R.W. Elliot

For British nephrologists of our generation the story of acute renal failure seemed to start in the London Blitz with the description of crush syndrome[1-5]. During the war years clinicians were also made aware of acute renal failure as a complication of septic abortion[6], black-water fever[7,8], fluid and electrolyte depletion[9,10] and injuries of various kinds not involving muscle crushing[11-14]. The search for a common pathogenesis was on. 'While the biochemical and renal changes associated with all these conditions are not identical, there is sufficient similarity to justify a search for a common aetiological basis' wrote Darmady and his colleagues in 1944. Maegraith, Havard and Parsons[15] went even further: '... we *must* remember the wide distribution of the syndrome: we *must* seek some factor which is common to all the many conditions in which it occurs'; the italics are ours but the earnestness of the search for a single explanation is in the original.

Since the end of World War 2 it has indeed become almost a tenet of nephrological faith that many forms of acute renal failure have a single pathogenisis. The mechanism postulated has varied from year to year; some became enshrined in the synonyms which gained at least fleeting acceptance: 'lower nephron nephrosis', 'acute tubular necrosis', 'shock kidney', 'renal anoxia', etc. As theory succeeded theory without any general agreement some of our colleagues suggested non-commital titles such as 'acute intrinsic renal failure'[16] or 'acute reversible intrinsic renal failure'[17] but they were not the neat, snappy phrases an advertising pundit would have chosen and they never quite caught on. 'Acute tubular necrosis' has remained the most popular title and has probably conditioned our thinking. We suppose that most medical students of the last quarter century have learned the sequence 'shock – renal vasoconstriction – anoxic damage to renal tubules – tubular necrosis and obstruction – prolonged oliguria : tubular regeneration – return of renal function'. Early in its life this theory was doubted by some clinicians who found it hard to accept that a process as gradual and presumably patchy as tubular regeneration could explain the sometimes abrupt onset of diuresis. However the studies of Bull, Joekes and Lowe[18] showed that restoration of glomerular filtration and tubular function lagged a long way behind the return of urine output to normal. We all recognise now that when oliguria officially ends, and urine volume exceeds 500 ml per 24 hours, the GFR is usually below 5 ml/min and it may still be less than 20 ml/min when the plasma urea is falling spontaneously and the patient on free fluid intake (Figure 2.1). Nonetheless much of the literature on acute renal failure in the last decade has been devoted to demolishing the central role of tubular necrosis and replacing it by some other mechanism[19].

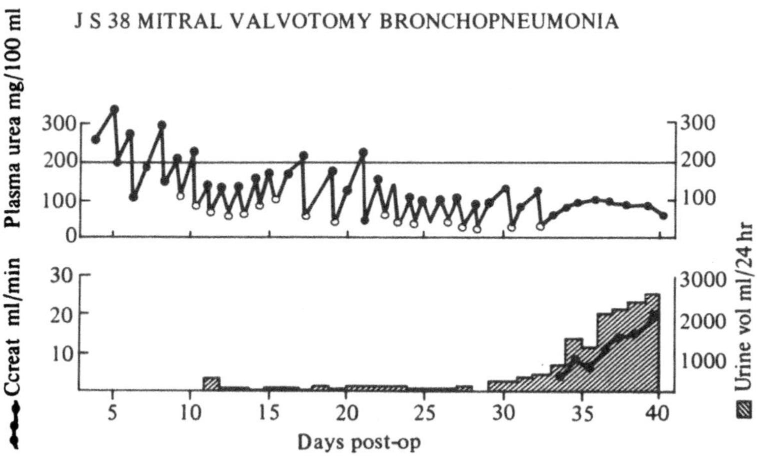

Figure 2.1 Clinical course of post-operative acute renal failure to illustrate the relationship between returning renal function and diuresis. (Reproduced by courtesy of Blackwell Scientific Publications, Oxford, England).

However the literature on acute renal failure did not begin in 1941. A great deal was written between the turn of the century and World War 2 about several forms of acute renal failure, notably those produced by mercuric chloride poisoning and transfusion reaction. We can only guess at the climate of medical opinion but it seems to us that investigators of that era looked for mechanisms specific to the condition they were studying and were hesitant to extrapolate their findings to other diseases. Some post-war authors have retained the same cautious attitude. Oliver[20] stated "There is no single 'cause' for oliguria but a great collection of causes". Muehrcke[21] commented that the aetiology was unknown in 30% of patients and multiple in many of the remainder and concluded '. . not only single mechanisms but combinations of mechanisms may explain the pathophysiology of acute renal failure'.

Diverse Causes

The cautious approach of Oliver[20] and Muehrcke[21] appeals to us because we are impressed by the diversity of the conditions which can cause acute renal failure; even a simplified account must include more than 20 major causes[22] and one major monograph describes 25 intrinsic renal diseases and lists over 70 drugs that have been incriminated[21]. This diversity is most obvious in the heterogeneous group labelled 'miscellaneous' in Tables 2.1 and 2.2 and called 'medical' by some authors. Post-partum renal failure is becoming a rarity in the U.K. and even the post traumatic variety may be on the wane in spite of our rising toll from traffic accidents; the 'miscellaneous' group is now becoming our major preoccupation (Table 2.3). It obviously comprises conditions of very different pathogenesis such as ureteric obstruction and renal arterial occlusion. It would not be surprising if there proved to be many other different pathways by which the various conditions in Table 2.3 produced the clinical syndrome of acute renal failure.

Table 2.1 Admission to the Acute Renal Failure Unit, Newcastle-upon-Tyne 1959–1972*

Complications of pregnancy		56
Complications of surgery		184
Complications of accidental trauma		62
Miscellaneous conditions		201
	Total	503

*This and subsequent tables exclude what is now our largest category of patients with acute renal failure – recipients of cadaver transplants

Table 2.2 'Miscellaneous' patients with acute renal failure admitted to Newcastle-upon-Tyne 1968–1972

Ureteric obstruction	17
Glomerulonephritis	11
Acute gn 3: Crescent gn 4	
D.L.E. 2: Other 2	
Infections	12
Fluid and electrolyte depletion	6
Nephrotoxins	5
Myocardial infarction	4
Pancreatitis	4
Myelomatosis	3
Others*	24
Total	86

*Including: Interstitial nephritis; Urate crystalluria; Transfusion reaction; Renal artery thrombosis; Hepatorenal syndrome; Analgesic nephropathy; Crohn's disease; Superior mesenteric artery thrombosis; Haematemesis; Microangiopathy

Table 2.3 Admission rate (patients per year) to the Acute Renal Failure Unit, Newcastle-upon-Tyne

Category	*1959–1963*	*1964–1967*	*1968–1972*
Pregnancy	6.0	3.5	2.2
Surgery	11.2	16.3	12.8
Trauma	5.2	5.0	3.2
Miscellaneous	11.0	15.0	17.2
Total	33.4	39.8	36.4

The trends shown in Table 2.3 are common in the U.K. and the U.S.A. but are not universal. In France[23-25] and many under-developed countries renal failure from pregnancy and abortion is still common. However even the apparently specific titles in Table 2.1 conceal many differences. The clinical course of acute renal failure following pre-eclampsia differs from that caused by abortion[26]. In the post-traumatic group, Whelton and

Donadio[27] have described a striking change in the cause and clinical picture between the wars in Korea and Vietnam. In the latter, early evacuation and resuscitation almost eliminated early acute renal failure due to shock. It was replaced by late-onset renal failure complicating sepsis in badly traumatised patients who would scarcely have survived with less active re-animation in the previous war; the course was prolonged and the prognosis poor. The same trends are discernible in civilian practice. The post-surgical group are a very mixed bunch. Many are elderly with the multiple pathology that accompanies old age (Table2.4). Their clinical course and prognosis vary according the primary operation (Table 2.5). The complication of surgery that precipitated acute renal failure cannot be identified in all (Table 2.6), in some there are several possible causes and in others an obvious accident that falls into none of our pathogenetic categories. The high mortality in patients with gastric surgery was associated with a high incidence of anastomotic rupture which appears to be both nephrotoxic and lethal whether or not it be accompanied by recognised shock.

Table 2.4 Age and sex of patients admitted to the Newcaste-upon-Tyne unit 1968–1972.

	Mean age	*Males (per cent)*
Pregnancy	29	0
Surgery	59	79
Trauma	35	81
Miscellaneous	52	59

An inconspicuous group in our Tables, but a much larger one in some other series, is nephrotoxic acute renal failure. The occurence of tubular necrosis in some nephrotoxic lesions has led to nephrotoxic and post-ischaemic acute renal failure being lumped together in many descriptions. This view has received support recently from the work of Hollenberg and his colleagues [28,29] who found similar derangements of renal blood flow distribution in both conditions. However Oliver, MacDowell and Tracy[30] showed that the extent of the necrosis and the damage to basement membranes were very different in the two conditions and that nephrotoxins damage the tubule at specific sites determined by their normal handling in the renal tubule. The ways in which drugs and poisons can damage the kidney are legion (Figure 2.2) and although they may not all be mediators of acute renal failure we think it is safer to consider nephrotoxic lesions separately. This is unfortunate since the most convenient animal model for acute renal failure is mercuric chloride nephropathy. Results have been extrapolated to the human lesion a little too readily.

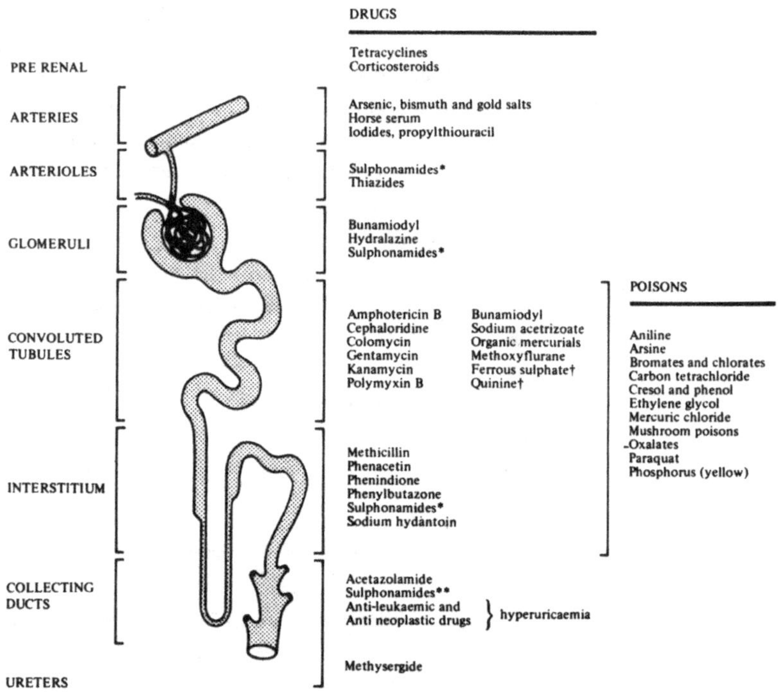

Figure 2.3 Sites at which drugs and poisons can damage the kidney. Modified from a diagram in Muehreke (1969). (From Kerr[22], Reproduced by courtesy of Blackwell Scientific Publications, Oxford, England).

Table 2.5 Relationship of survival rate to original operation site in 160 patients treated at Newcastle-upon-Tyne

Operation Site	*Number*	*Mortality rate (per cent)*
Stomach and duodenum	29	72
Biliary tract	13	54
Other abdominal	40	58
Genito urinary	29	41
Gynaecological	15	20
Cardiac, vascular	27	52
Miscellaneous	7	57
Total	160	52

Table 2.6 Identified causes of acute renal failure in 102 post-operative patients (Elliott and Kerr, 1967)[159]

*Shock – hypotension recorded	35
Fluid and electrolyte imbalance	22
Infection	15
No cause identified	30

*Includes four transfusion reactions

Unifying Concepts

Although we are sceptical of one pathogenisis for acute renal failure following most of its many causes there must be a limit to the ways in which the kidney can respond to injury. Common links in the chain of causation must be sought since it is at these points that we are most likely to be successful in breaking the chain and preventing acute renal failure. Until recently there has been almost universal agreement on the initial insult – shock and temporary renal ischaemia – and controversy has centred on the cause of the prolonged oliguria. Recent speculation on the roles of renin and disseminated intravascular coagulation has thrown the whole field wide open once again.

The Initial Insult

Tubular blockage

The first explanation put forward for the oliguria of acute renal failure was blockage of the tubules by casts. The idea was suggested by the numerous pigmented casts found in the kidney after fatal transfusion accidents and it was apparently confirmed by the work of Baker and Dodds[31] who showed that intravenous haemoglobin produced acute renal failure in rabbits only if the urine was acid and had a high solute content. In these circumstances they found that haemoglobin was precipitated *in vitro*. In an instructive case report[32] Witts described the application of this theory to a woman with oliguria following a transfusion reaction. She was given intravenous fluid and potassium citrate to reduce the concentration and acidity of her urine. She died suddenly in the early diuretic phase from what sounds like a hyperkalaemic cardiac arrest and was waterlogged at autopsy.

The early papers on crush syndrome emphasised the pigmented myoglobin casts in the tubules and suggested that these might be the primary cause of the anuria. Bywaters and Stead[33] were unable to produce acute renal failure in rabbits by muscle damage unless they injected myoglobin (not present in any quantity in normal rabbit muscle) and acidified the urine (they did not try the two manoeuvres separately). However they discarded the cast blockage theory as they found casts to be an inconstant feature of the renal pathology of crush syndrome, at least in two-dimensional histological studies[7]. Ayer and Gauld[34] rejected cast blockage as the cause of oliguria in transfusion reaction since they found cast formation at least as prominent in infants with obstructive jaundice without renal dysfunction. Some patients and dogs had more evidence of tubular necrosis than of pigment casts after transfusion reaction[35] and there was little correlation between urinary acidity, solute content or the severity of haemoglobinuria and the development of acute renal failure in blackwater fever[8].

Acute renal failure can be produced by injecting haemoglobin or methaemoglobin into dogs and rabbits or by producing muscle damage in the rat with intramuscular glycerol; cast formation is a prominent feature of all such models. Harrison and his colleagues[36] found a good correlation between the number of casts formed, judged by microdissection, and the depression of GFR. They observed cast formation before any reduction in renal plasma flow and attributed oliguria to the viscocity of tubular fluid during the formation of casts. Mason, Teschan and Muirhead[37] observed dilation of tubules proximal to casts beginning 30 mins after the induction of acute renal failure in rats by methaemoglobin and this preceded prolonged reduction in renal blood flow. Jaenike[38] found a mixed picture in the same model; some tubules were shown by micropuncture to have raised intraluminar pressure indicating obstruction, while others were collapsed suggesting a primary reduction in GFR. Ruiz-Guinazu, Coelho and Paz[39] noted a transient dilation of proximal tubules after injection of methaemoglobin and a few remained dilated above casts. However the majority of the proximal tubules soon became collapsed and they concluded that obstruction was not of major importance Oken, Arce and Wilson[40] found no rise in proximal tubular pressure and they were able to wash the agglutinating sludge out of the tubules with a pressure of only 15–20 cm water which was well below the presumed filtration pressure in the rat. They concluded that a fall in GFR caused cast formation rather than vice versa. However they had difficulty in dislodging fully formed casts from renal tubules suggesting that these could have a role in maintaining oliguria even if they do not cause it. Flamembaum[41] has reviewed the confusing literature on these animal models and concludes that cast formation is not the primary event.

However a primary role for tubular blockage by casts is still postulated by some authors in a few special circumstances. In myelomatosis acute renal failure is believed to occur through at least five different mechanisms – infiltration, hyperuricaemia, hypercalcaemia, hyperviscocity and blockage by casts of Bence-Jones protein – of which the last is much the commonest[42]. If powerful diuretics really do reverse acute renal failure at the onset stage as many have claimed[43,44] and if they act partly or wholly by preventing tubular blockage with cellular debris or casts, this is one situation in which they ought to be dramatically effective. It is the only one in which we have been convinced that diuretics unequivocally altered the course of acute renal failure (Figure 2.3).

Tubular blockage may be the basis of acute renal failure following pyelography in dehydrated patients; pyelographic media can precipitate Tamm–Horsfall mucoprotein *in vitro*[45].

Finally, tubular casts must still be considered as a cause of acute renal failure complicating muscle injury. Myoglobin casts in the urine and in the kidney are a prominent feature of acute renal failure following heat stress and unaccustomed exercise[46-49] episodes of paroxysmal myoglobinuria[50-54], McArdle's Disease[55] seasnake poisoning[56], hornet stings[57], arterial embolism[58], electrical burns[59], carbon monoxide or sedative poisoning[60-62] and dermatomyositis[63]. Shock or/and intravascular coagulation are features of some of these syndromes but some patients appear to develop renal failure with no other precipitant than unaccustomed exercise and muscle damage[49]. The young serviceman shown in Figure 2.4 was subjected to heavy exercise on the vaulting horse soon after enlistment. He felt unwell and reported sick but was reassured and allowed to continue exercise. His subsequent acute renal failure had no obvious precipitating cause apart from the muscle damage in his thighs.

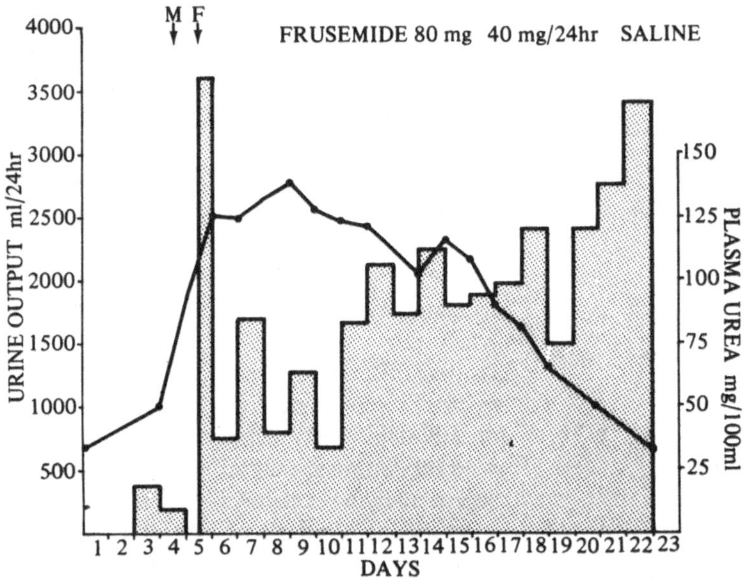

Figure 2.3 Relief of oliguria following injection of frusemide (F) in a patient with myelomatosis excreting Bence–Jones Protein. Previous injection of mannitol (M) was unsuccessful

Since the fall in GFR, proteinuria and cast excretion that accompany strenuous exercise are attributed to renal vasoconstriction, muscle injury may not be the only factor in this type of acute renal failure, but it is hard to escape the conviction that myoglobin excretion is 'bad for the kidneys'.

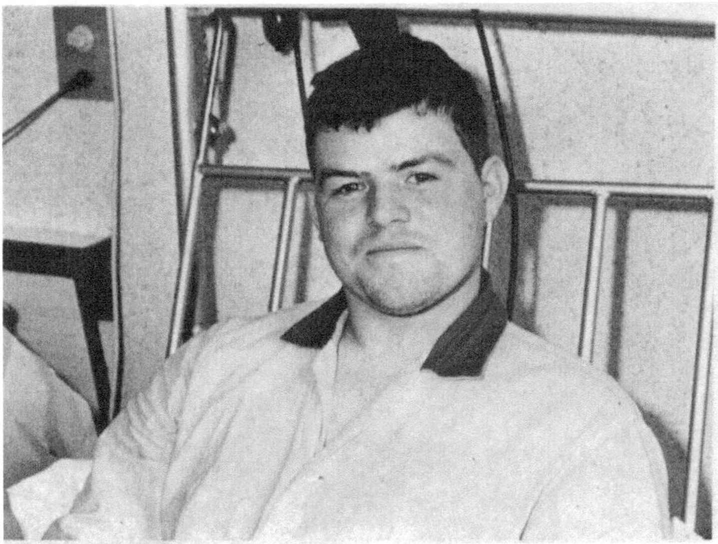

Figure 2.4 Fit and muscular young man who developed acute renal failure following strenuous exercise to which he was unaccustomed and which produced pain in the thigh muscles.

Cortical ischaemia

Since Maegraith, Havard and Parsons[15] postulated that shock was the common mediator of most forms of acute renal failure the concept has been almost universally accepted. The work of Trueta and his colleagues[64] provided an impressive animal model (Figure 2.5), and subsequent investigators have provided many others (see Flamembaum[65] for review). The cortical ischaemia during shock is not always as uniform as Figure 2.5 suggests. Injection studies with thioflavine S[30] show patchy ischaemia in several nephrotoxic lesions and a similar pattern has been found by corrosion techniques in shock kidney[66]. As Brod[67] points out these studies show the renal circulation at only one moment in time; it is conceivable that the maximum vasoconstriction affects different parts of the cortex from hour to hour or minute to minute, protecting it from the worst effects of ischaemia. A fall in GFR occurs so early in experimental acute renal failure that it is almost certainly a direct result of this renal vasoconstriction[40,65].

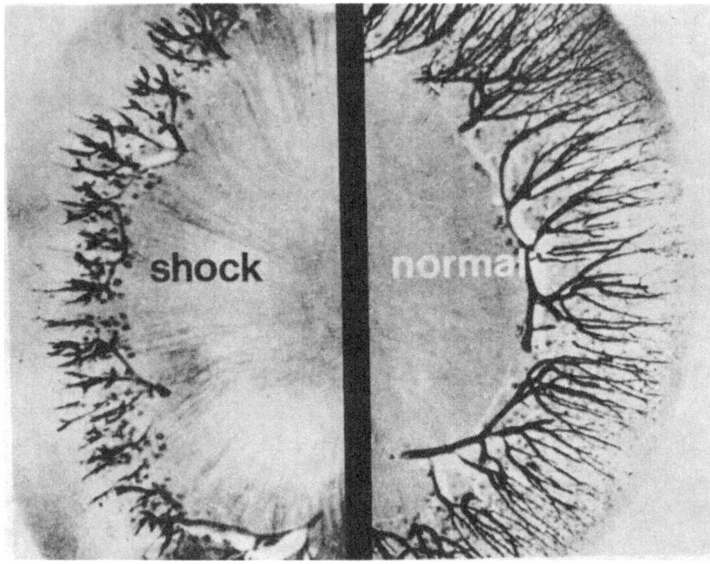

Figure 2.5 Cortical ischaemia produced by shock. Modified from Trueta *et al.*[64]

The work of Trueta and his colleagues[64] suggested that sympathetic stimulation might be responsible for renal vasoconstriction and both the pattern of cortical ischaemia found in acute renal failure and oliguria can be reproduced by injecting adrenaline into the renal artery [69,70]. Grandchamp, Ayer and Truniger[71] were able to prevent cortical ischaemia in hypotensive dogs by alpha-adrenergic blockade with phenoxybenzamine or phentolamine but not with other vasodilators. However they also showed that hypotension produced its characteristic changes in renal perfusion after acute or chronic denervation of the kidney by autotransplantation and concluded that circulating catecholamines must be more important than sympathetic nerves[72]. Their conclusion is backed up by a good deal of clinical experience; acute renal failure can occur after renal transplantation in response to shock or sepsis. Recently it has been suggested again that renin and angiotensin may be responsible for the initial renal ischaemia[19,65]. However renin-depleted rats who are resistant to the development of acute renal failure still suffer initial cortical ischaemia; it is of shorter duration and causes less damage than in the controls suggesting that if renin plays a role in producing acute renal failure it is at a later stage[73,74].

There are few opportunities for studying renal haemodynamics in man at the onset of acute renal failure but a few high-risk groups have been investigated. In shocked patients with myocardial infarction Hutton and his colleagues[75] found that renal plasma flow was reduced to about 40 per cent of normal and this was accompanied by oliguria and passage of urine with an osmolality close to that of plasma. Unfortunately they omitted to say whether these patients subsequently remained in acute renal failure or recovered when their blood pressure rose. After severe trauma mainly from gunshots, Rosenberg and his colleagues[76] found a reduction in renal plasma flow and a greater reduction in GFR which persisted after restoration of blood volume. Patients who subsequently developed acute renal failure had more severe depression of blood flow, lower GFR and higher renal vascular resistance than their fellows. Sepsis on the other hand appeared to produce renal vasodilatation and paradoxical polyuria[77]. These studies leave unanswered the question that was asked as soon the role of vasoconstriction was postulated in the 1940s; if shock causes renal vasoconstriction and vasoconstriction causes acute renal failure why do so many patients recover from shock without renal damage? Several shocked patients with gastrointestinal haemorrhage are treated each week in Newcastle but only one appears in Table 2.3. Is it solely a question of how long the vasoconstriction lasts or are there complementary factors which help to produce renal damage? Two possible 'co-factors' in damaging the kidney are renin hypersecretion and disseminated intravascular coagulation; each has its enthusiastic proponents.

Mediators of Renal Damage

Renin-Angiotensin

In 1945 Goormaghtigh[78] examined the afibrillar cells of the juxtaglomerular apparatus from patients with crush syndrome and commented 'In no other pathological condition yet examined is the hypertrophy and granularity . . . so marked'. He postulated that a '. . . vasopressive substance is liberated in excess and causes a persistent spasm at the vascular pole of the glomerular tufts'. His theory lay dormant for 20 years but was revived to explain the effects of hydration on the development of acute renal failure in rats. Thiel and his colleagues[158] found that dehydration greatly increased the susceptibility of rats to myoglobin-induced renal failure and attributed this to reduction in plasma volume. To exclude the possibility that hyperconcentration of the urine was the predisposing factor they repeated their studies in dehydrated rats with diabetes insipidus and showed that continuing urine flow did not protect them[79]. Loading with saline to deplete the rats of renin largely protected them from the development of acute renal failure, despite initial vasoconstriction[73,80], and a high sodium diet had a similar protective effect[81]. These experiments do not prove that renin is responsible for the changes in susceptibility and other mediators such as prostaglandins were suggested[82]. However the case for renin was strengthened when it was shown that plasma renin and angiotensin are elevated early in the course of acute renal failure and slowly subside as renal function returns[83-85]. To clinch the argument it would be necessary to show that blocking the effect of renin or angiotensin prevented acute renal failure without manipulating plasma volume etc. In rats, immunisation against renin failed to protect against myoglobinuria[41]. However Brown and his colleagues[84] suggested that the accumulation of renin and eventually of angiotensin 2 might be confined to the kidney with little change in circulating levels of these hormones and by implication the most important renin may be inaccessible to the antibody. Subsequently they showed that rats immunised against angiotensin 2 were protected against myoglobunuric acute renal failure[86]. On the other hand[68] Matthews, Morgan and Johnston could demonstrate no protection in similar experiments. The case for a major role of renin has been expounded by Flamembaum[65] and in the Lancet[19] while some of the objections are set out in the British Medical Journal[87].

Disseminated Intravascular Coagulation

There is no doubt about the importance of intravascular coagulation in the haemolytic uraemic syndrome of children and adults[88,89] in 'Robson's syndrome' of early post-partum renal failure[90-93] and in other microangiopathies. Thrombosis in vessels from the arcuate arteries to the afferent arterioles causes glomerular infarction and patchy cortical necrosis, thrombi are present in glomerular capillaries and the changes in coagulation factors, platelet count and red cell morphology bear witness to the presence of intravascular fibrin[94]. Vassali and Richet[95] presented the case for intravascular coagulation as the cause of bilateral cortical necrosis in which some of these changes in the peripheral blood may be observed. A human counterpart of the Shwartzman reaction is now recognised[96].

On the other hand there has been a general reluctance to accept intravascular coagulation as a factor in the commoner types of reversible acute renal failure. From the earliest descriptions of renal morphology it has been emphasised that the glomeruli, although bloodless and shrunken[20] are essentially normal on light and electron microscopy[97–99]. However few investigators have seen the earliest changes in acute renal failure in the human. Sevitt[100] who studied burned patients found extensive glomerular thrombosis in eight, five of whom died between 24 and 48 hours of injury and all of whom had tubular necrosis. He concluded that glomerular thrombosis was a transient phenomenon since he rarely encountered it in patients dying at a later stage and without giving any reasons he stated that 'It is unlikely that (it) plays a significant part in the pathogenisis of tubular necrosis'. Quite different conclusions were drawn by Clarkson *et al.*[101] who studied biopsies taken from 4 to 42 (median 16) days after the onset of oliguria. Like previous authors they found that glomeruli (with one exception) were normal on light microscopy but 'electron microscopy revealed lesions unsuspected on light microscopy'. These consisted of epithelial swelling, capillary narrowing and the presence of fibrin-like material in the capillaries and Bowman's spaces. They regarded these lesions as sufficiently severe to play an important part in the production of necrosis in tubules supplied by post-glomerular capillaries from the affected glomeruli. Their patients had elevated fibrin degradation products in serum during the oliguric phase and in urine at the onset of diuresis, a finding confirmed by many other studies[102–104].

Disseminated intravascular coagulation (DIC) is now recognised as a syndrome of wide distribution in medicine[105]. Pregnancy, which impairs the activity of the reticuloendothelial system is an important predisposing cause (Figure 2.6). Florid DIC with characteristic changes in the blood occurs in septic abortion [106] and this is the commonest cause of the syndrome in the renal unit[25,107,108]. Even clean, therapeutic abortion can cause defibrination[109,110] and pre-eclampsia is another recognised cause[111–113]. In acute renal failure following conditions other than pregnancy, typical changes in the coagulation system are seldom found; in anything plasma fibrinogen is raised and the blood hypercoaguable[101,114]. However this does not exclude the possibility that defibrination occurred before the onset of acute renal failure and indeed there is every reason to believe that this frequently occurs. Intravascular coagulation is a characteristic feature of shock[115], sepsis[116-119], malignant malaria[120-122], pancreatitis[123], mercurial poisoning[124], some drug reactions[125] and many other conditions that predispose to acute renal failure.

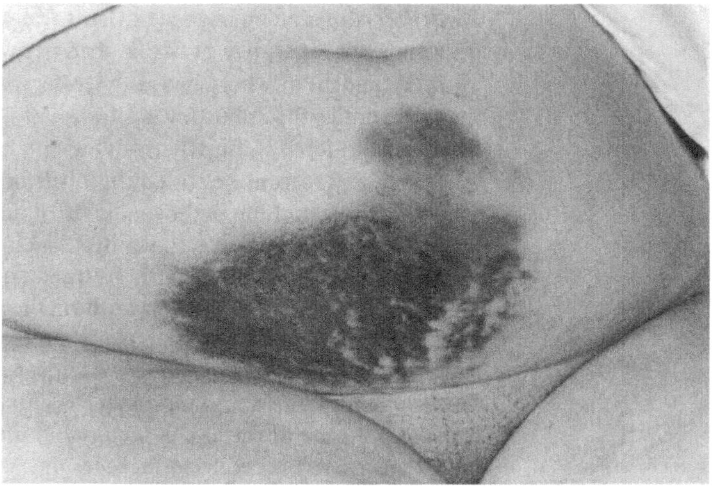

Figure 2.6 'DIC⇒ARF'
Bruising at the site of 'gentle massage of the uterus' in a patients with disseminated intravascular coagulation causing hypofibrinogenaemia and acute renal failure

One of the problems of investigating the role of DIC is the high fibrinolytic activity of the kidney[126,127] which may remove all trace of thrombi that have nonetheless caused ischaemic damage. The transient nature of intra-renal thrombosis has been demonstrated after renal arterial occlusion[128] and the injection of procoagulant substances into the renal arteries[129]. However microthrombi can be found in the renal circulation of many patients at autopsy if sought sufficiently hard[130]. If they are not extensive enough to occlude vessels at any stage in their development they may still be important in producing arteriolar spasm by the release of vasoconstrictor substances[129,131]. Radiofibrinogen studies show that excessive thrombosis is occurring somewhere in the circulation even after the development of acute renal failure[132], so this mechanism could even play a role in the continuing oliguria.

Cause of Prolonged Oliguria

During the onset of acute renal failure renal function seems to change from a state of rapidly reversible impairment, characterised by some concentrating ability, to one of temporary irreversibility when urinary osmolality is close to that of plasma[133]. Thereafter oliguria persists for days or weeks. The cause of this continuing oliguria has been hotly debated for a quarter century.

Renal Oedema

In 1945 Peters[134] propounded the theory that increased pressure from the swollen kidney inside its restraining capsule prevented glomerular filtration by hydrostatic pressure. The theory was apparently well accepted at the time for the article quotes an editor of the Lancet as stating 'You are no doubt right in urging that the raised intrarenal pressure is the basis of the transfusion and crush kidney and that this can best be treated by decapsulation. The treatments you recommend – decapsulation, diuretics and pressor drugs – are now widely used separately or in combination'. Abeshouse[135] reviewed an extensive literature on decapsulation and added ten cases of his own; the reported success rate in some forms of acute renal failure was over 80 per cent but the observations were uncontrolled and selected like all published case reports, and the operation fell into disrepute with the introduction of conservative treatment. Direct measurement of intrarenal pressure in experimental acute renal failure[136] and the measurement of wedged renal vein pressure in patients[137] showed no increase in pressure in the renal venules and, by implication, none in the interstitium. Some authors have been impressed with the incidence and severity of oedema of the interstitium in acute renal failure, as shown by renal biopsy[97,155] but others have found it an inconstant part of the pathology[21,28]. The theory has quietly died but never been decently buried.

Leakage of Filtrate

The leakage of filtrate through damaged epithelium or breaks in the basement membrane was the theory favoured by Oliver, MacDowell and Tracy[30] after their microdissection studies. It was supported by indirect evidence from the studies on nephrotoxic acute renal failure by Sims and colleagues[138] and more directly by the micropuncture studies of Bank, Mutz and Avendjian[139] who observed the excessive re-absorption of lissamine green from still functioning proximal tubules. However, with one exception, subsequent micropuncture studies have failed to confirm this finding even when carried out at a time when tubular necrosis is obvious[140]. The back diffusion theory his therefore out of favour[65].

Tubular Necrosis

Bywaters and Dible[7] described the lesion in crush syndrome as follows: 'The proximal convoluted tubules are the seat of an intense catarrh, so that the lumina are filled with detritus and masses . . . (which) . . . appear to be the remains of epithelial cells . . . The wide ascending limb of Henle's loop and the second convoluted tubule show the most severe damage'. Subsequent authors disagreed about the site of maximum damage; Lucke[141] placed it in the distal tubule while Sevitt[100] described proximal and distal tubular necrosis as separate lesions which seldom coexisted in the same patient. There was no general agreement either about the way in which tubular necrosis caused oliguria. Bywaters and Dible[7] favoured leakage of filtrate because they did not think a sufficiently high proportion of the tubules were affected for obstruction to be an acceptable explanation. Oliver, MacDowell and Tracy[30] drew the same conclusion for different reasons. Their microdissection studies showed that the tubular lesions were much more widespread than appeared on two-dimensional histology. Meroney and Rubini[143] interpreted their functional studies as indicating that the little urine passed during the oliguric phase was derived from surviving normal nephrons while the majority were blocked by debris. On the other hand Finckh, Jeremy and Whyte[144] and Olsen[146] concluded that tubular necrosis was too inconstant and often inconspicuous a feature to be the explanation of oliguria in acute renal failure. Their view was based on light or electron microscopy but Darmady and Stranack[157] also found some patients without tubular lesions on microsdissection. In rats wiht mercuric chloride poisoning, Di Bona and colleagues[156] showed that the oliguric phase could be abolished by saline loading in spite of the development of tubular necrosis as severe as that in the control (oliguric) rats.

The present concensus of opinion is therefore that tubular necrosis is not the major cause of oliguria in acute renal failure[65]. However we feel that its importance is being dismissed a little too readily. Henry, Lane and Kashgarian[146] while attributing oliguria to reduced cortical flow also demonstrated that obstruction of the distal tubule was probably a factor in prolonging oliguria in the rat. The evidence, quoted above, that sludge and obstructing casts can be dislodged by pressure below filtration pressure is less convincing in the light of new evidence that filtration pressure is lower than previously supposed[147]. We find it hard to accept that this striking histological lesion often showing total disruption of the tubular lining is without functional significance.

Prolonged Cortical Ischaemia

Sevitt[142] found tubular necrosis in so many patients dying without acute renal failure that he discarded the theories which rested on tubular damage as the mediator of oliguria. In their place he proposed a theory that the persistent reduction of GFR was due to prolonged renal vasoconstriction. This concept has gradually gained acceptance and is now orthodox[65]. The first measurements of renal blood flow during the oliguric phase showed that they averaged about 40 per cent of normal[148-150]. This was scarcely low enough to account for oliguria, particularly as occasional patients had normal renal blood flow[150]. Reduced renal blood flow of this order is compatible with good renal output in chronic renal disease but in this situation blood flow is normally distributed between the cortex and medulla[28]. In acute renal failure selective reduction of cortical flow is shown by angiography[28,151] by xenon washout curves[152] and by poor bleeding at open biopsy[28]. Direct measurements of intraglomerular pressure in the rat with myoglobin-induced renal failure suggest that the resistance is mainly in the afferent arteriole[74]. There was a very close correlation between cortical blood flow and GFR and both of these parameters were improved in parallel by prior saline loading.

If renal vasoconstriction does indeed persist for weeks, what is the stimulus? One possibility is a viscious cycle involving continuous release of renin which perpetuates the spasm that produced it; another is cellular swelling produced by the initial ischaemia[19]. Although epithelial swelling has been shown in glomerular capillaries[101,153], the afferent arteriole has not so far been incriminated. The vasoconstrictor substances released during intravascular thrombosis[131] are a third possibility. The theory of nervous of humoral vasoconstriction would acquire a firmer foundation, and the therapy of acute renal failure a revolutionary change, if it could be demonstrated that any vasodilator substance rapidly reversed the oliguria; no such demonstration has been forthcoming.

The Late Recovery Phase

After acute renal failure the GFR returns to about 70 or 80 per cent of normal, on average (see Kerr[22] for review). This is about the same level of function that follows nephrectomy for unilateral disease suggesting that about half the nephrons are lost during an episode of acute tubular necrosis. The graphic descriptions of tubular repair, kinking and blockage by Oliver[20] provide a ready explanation.

Conclusion

If this account seems confused and indecisive it accurately reflects the state of mind of the authors after reviewing the literature. Jaenike[38] described micropuncture studies on the rat in acute renal failure which revealed obstructed tubules, tubules with no GFR and no obstruction and many intermediate values 'indicating that both obstruction and failure of filtration were operative'. If you find that complexity in a stereotyped animal model it would be a bold man who dogmatised about the pathogenisis of acute renal failure in our typical Saturday lunch-time admission with sclerotic renal arteries, sunken orbits but swollen legs, an assortment of gram-negative and gram-positive organisms in his blood stream, with high plasma renin, angiotensin, catecholamines, fibrin degradation products, gentamycin, cephaloridine and frusemide levels and low plasma volume, blood pressure, platelet count and morale. We are not that bold.

References

1. Beall, D., Bywaters, E.G.L., Belsey, R.H.R. and Miles, J.A.R. (1941) 'A case of crush injury with renal failure'. *Brit. Med. J.* 1, 432–434
2. Bywaters, E.G.L. and Beall, D. (1941). Crush injuries with impairment or renal function. *Brit. Med. J.*, 1, 427–432
3. Longland, C.J. and Murray, J. (1941). A case of recovery from crush syndrome. *Lancet*, 2, 158–159
4. Maitland, A.I.L. (1941). A case of crush injury with recovery *Lancet*, 2, 446–448

5. Mayon-White, R. and Solandt, O.M. (1941). A case of limb compression ending fatally in uraemia. *Brit. Med. J.*, **1**, 434–435
6. Bratton, A.B. (1941). Anuria with casts not associated with transfusion. *Lancet*, **1**, 345–346
7. Bywaters, E.G.L. and Dible.,J.H. (1942). The renal lesion in traumatic anuria. *J. Path. Bact.*, **54**, 111–119
8. Maegraith, B. (1944). Blackwater fever anuria. *Trans. Roy. Soc. Trop. Med. Hygiene*, **38**, 1–17
9. Nichol, B.M. (1940). The renal changes in alkalosis. *Quart. J. Med.*, **9**, 91–105
10. McLetchie, N.G.B. (1943). Renal lesions in a case of excessive vomiting. *J. Path. and Bact.*, **55**, 17–22
11. Glen, A.M. (1941). Temporary vascular occlusion ending fatally in uraemia. *Brit. Med. J.*, **2**, 875–876
12. Bywaters, E.G.L. and Belsey, R.H.R. (1942). Discussion on the effects on the kidney of trauma to parts other than the urinary tract including crush syndrome. *Proc. Roy. Soc. Med.*,**35**, 321–328
13. Cumings, J.N. (1942). The occurrence of uraemia in head injury and the histological features of the renal lesions. *J. Path. and Bact.* **54**, 532–533
14. Darmady, E.M., Siddons, A.H.M., Corson, T.C., Langton, C.D., Vitek, Z., Badenoch, A.W. and Scott, J.C. (1944). Traumatic uraemia, reports on eight cases. *Lancet*, **2**, 809–812
15. Maegraith, B.G., Havard, R.E. and Parsons, D.S. (1945). Renal syndrome of wide distribution induced possibly by renal anoxia. *Lancet*,**2**, 293–296
16. Shaldon, S. (1966). Acute renal failure. (R. Daly and H.G. Miller, editors) *Progress in Clinical Medicine*, 5th edn, p. 233–245
17. Luke, R.G. and Kennedy, A.C. (1967). Prevention and early management of acute renal failure. *Postgrad. Med.J.*, **43**, 280–289
18. Bull, G.M., Joekes, A.M. and Lowe, K.G. (1950). Renal function studies in acute tubular necrosis. *Clin. Sci.*, **9**, 379–404
19. Acute renal failure, (1973). *Lancet*, **2**, 134–135
20. Oliver, J. (1953). Correlations of structure and function and mechanism of recovery in acute tubular necrosis. *Amer. J. Med.*, **15**, 535–557
21. Muehrcke, R.C. (1969). *Acute renal failure: Diagnosis and Management.* (St Louis: Mosby)
22. Kerr, D.N.S. (1973). Acute Renal Failure. *Renal Disease*, (D.A.K. Black, editor, Oxford: Blackwell) 417–461
23. Derot, M., Legrain, M., Guedon, J., Pignard, P. and Roy, J.L. (1966) L'Insufficance rénale aiguë 'Post abortum'. A propos de 215 observations. *Presse Médicale*, **74**, 1579–1584
24. Legrain, M., Baguet, J.C., Didon, D. and Beaufils, F. (1970). Prognostic et traitment de l'insufficance rénale aiguë post abortum. *Presse Médicale*, **78**, 1565–1570
25. Beruard, M., Ducluzeau, R., Zech, P.Y., Traeger, J. (1973). Coagulation intra-vasculaire disseminée et insufficance rénale aiguë. A propos de trente observations. *Lyon Médicale*, **229**, 771–784
26. Elliott, R.W., Ashcroft, R., Clarkson, B.A., Kerr, D.N.S. and Robson, A. (1964). Long-term follow-up of renal function following acute renal failure complicating pregnancy. *Proc. Europ. Dialysis and Transplant. Ass.*, **1**, 107–112

27. Whelton, A. and Donadio, J.V. (1969). Post-traumatic acute renal failure in Vietnam. *Johns Hopkins Med. J.*, **124**, (2), 95–105
28. Hollenberg, N.K., Epstein, M., Rosen, S.M., Basch, R.I., Oken, D.E. and Merrill, J.P. (1968). Acute oliguric renal failure in man: evidence for preferential cortical ischemia. *Medicine*, **47**, 455–474
29. Hollenberg, N.K., Adams, D.F., Oken, D.E., Abrams, H.L. and Merrill, J.P. (1970). Acute renal failure due to nephrotoxins. Renal hemodynamic and angiographic studies in man. *New Eng. J. Med.*, **282**, 1329–1334
30. Oliver, J., MacDowell, M. and Tracy, A. (1951). The pathogenesis of acute renal failure with traumatic and toxic injury. Renal ischemia, nephrotoxic damage and the ischemuric episode. *J. Clin. Invest.*, **30**, 1305–1351
31. Baker, S.J. and Dodds, E.C. (1925). Obstruction of renal tubules during the excretion of hemoglobin. *Brit. J. Exp. Path.*, **6**, 247–260
32. Witts, L.J. (1929). A note on blood transfusion with an account of a fatal reaction. *Lancet*, **1**, 1297–1299
33. Bywaters, E.G.L. and Stead, J.K. (1944). The production of renal failure following injection of solutions containing myohemoglobin. *Quart. J. Exp. Physiol.*, **33**, 53–70
34. Ayer, G.D. and Gauld, A.G. (1942). Uremia following blood transfusion The nature and the significance of the renal changes. *Arch. Path.*, **33**, 513–532
35. DeGowin, E.L., Warner, E.D. and Randall, W.L. (1938). Renal insufficiency from blood transfusion. *Arch. Inter Med.*, **61**, 609–630
36. Harrison, H.E., Bunting, H., Ordway, N.K. and Albrink, W.S. (1947). The pathogenisis of the renal injury produced in the dog by hemoglobin or methemoglobin. *J. Exp. Med.* **86**, 339–356
37. Mason, A.D., Teschan, P.E. and Muirhead, E.E. (1963). Studies in acute renal failure. 3. Renal histologic alterations in acute renal failure in the rat. *J. Surg.Res.* **3**, 450–456
38. Jaenike, J.R. (1969). Micropuncture study of methemoglobin induced acute renal failure in the rat. *J. Lab. Clin. Med.*, **73**, 459–468
39. Ruiz, Guinazu, A., Coelho, J.B. and Paz, R.A. (1967). Methemoglobin induced acute renal failure in the rat. *Nephron*, **4**, 257–275
40. Oken, D.E., Arce, M.L. and Wilson, D.R. (1966). Glycerol induced hemoglobinuric acute renal failure in the rat. 1. Micropuncture study of the development of oliguria. *J. Clin. Inv.*, **45**, 724–735
41. Flamembaum, W., Kotchen, T.A. and Oken, D.E. (1972). Effect of renin immunization on mercuric chloride and glycerol-induced renal failure. *Kidney International*, **1**, 406–412
42. Martinez-Maldonado, M., Yium, J., Suki, W.N. and Eknoyan, G. (1971). Renal complications in multiple myeloma. *J. Chron. Dis.*, **24**, 221–237
43. Bailey, R.R., Natale, R., Turnbull, D.I. and Linton, A.L. (1973). Protective effect of frusemide in acute tubular necrosis and acute renal failure. *Clin. Sci. Molec. Med.*, **45**, 1–17
44. Kjellstrand, C.M. (1973). Ethacrynic acid in acute tubular necrosis. *Nephron*, **9**, 337–348
45. Schwartz, R.H., Berdon, W.E., Wagner, J., Becker, J. and Baker, D.H. (1970). Tamm-Horsfall urinary mucoprotein precipitation by urographic contrast agents: *in vitro* studies. *Amer. J. Roentgenol. Radium Therapy, and Nucl. Med.*, **108**, 698–701

46. Schrier, R.W., Henderson, H.S., Tisher, G.C. and Tannen, R.L. (1967). Nephropathy associated with heat stress and exercise. *Annal. Inter. Med.*, **67**, 356–376
47. Schrier, R.W., Hano, J., Keller, H.I., Finkel, R.M., Gilliland, P.F., Cirksena, W.J. and Teschan, P.E. (1970). Renal metabolic and circulatory responses to heat and exercise. *Annal. Inter. Med.*, **73**, 213–223
48. Vertel, R.M. and Knochel, J.P. (1967). Acute renal failure due to heat injury. *Amer. J. Med.*, **43**, 435–451
49. Hamilton, R.W., Gardner, L.B., Penn, A.S. and Goldberg, M. (1972). Acute tubular necrosis caused by exercise-induced myoglobinuria. *Annal, Inter. Med.*, **77**, 77–82
50. Tavill, A.S., Evanson, J.M., Baker, S.B. de C. and Hewitt, V. (1964). Idiopathic paroxysmal myoglobinuria with acute renal failure and hypercalcemia. *New Eng J.Med.*, **271**, 283–287
51. Goldberg, W.M., and Chakrabarti, S.G. (1966). Idiopathic paroxysmal myoglobinuria with transient renal failure. *Can. Med. Assn.J.*, **94**, 681–683
52. Quinn, M., Wolf, J.S. and Lester, J. (1966). Relationship of acute renal failure to muscle necrosis. *New York State J. of Med.*, **66**, 400–403
53. Leonard, C.D. and Eichner, E.R. (1970). Acute renal failure and transient hypercalcemia in idiopathic rhabdomyolysis. *J. Amer. Med. Assn.* **211**, 1539–1540
54. Kagen, L.J. (1970). Immunogluorescent demonstration of myoglobin in the kidney. *Amer. J. Med.*, **48**, 649–653
55. Grünfeld, J.-P., Ganeval, D., Chanard, J., Fardau, M. and Dreyfus, J. -C. (1972). Acute renal failure in McArdle's disease. Report of two cases. *New Eng. J. Med.*, **286**, 1237–1241
56. Sitprija, V., Sribhibhadh, R. and Benyajati, C. (1971). Hemodialysis in poisoning by sea-snake venom. *Brit. Med. J.*, **3**, 218–219
57. Shilkin, K.B., Chen, B.T.M. and Khoo, O.T. (1972). Rhabdomyolysis caused by Hornet venom. *Brit. Med. J.*, **1**, 156–157
58. Haimovici, H. (1970). Arterial embolism, myoglobinuria and renal tubular necrosis. *Archio. Surg.*, **100**, 639–645
59. Platts, M.M. and Rozner, L. (1966). Survival after high-tension electrical burns complicated by acute tubular necrosis. *Brit. Med. J.*, **1**, 781–782
60. Loughridge, L.W., Leader, L.P. and Bowen, D.A.L. (1958). Acute renal failure due to muscle necrosis in carbon monoxide poisoning. *Lancet*, **2**, 349–351
61. Linton, A.L., Adams, J.H. and Lawson, D.H. (1968). Muscle necrosis and acute renal failure in carbon monoxide poisoning. *Postgrad. Med. J.* **44**, 338–342
62. Schreiber, S.N., Leibowitz, M.R. and Bernstein, L.H. (1972). Limb compression and renal impairment (crush syndrome) following narcotic and sedative overdose. *J. Bone and Joint Surgery.*, **54A**, 1683–1692
63 Kessler, E., Weinberger, I. and Rosenfeld, J.B. (1972). Myoglobinuric acute renal failure in a case of dermatomyositis. *Israel J. Med. Sci.*, **8**, 978–983
64. Trueta, J., Barclay, A.E., Daniel, P.M., Franklin, K.J. and Pritchard, M.M.L. (1947). *Studies of the Renal Circulation.* (Oxford: Blackwell)
65. Flamembaum, W. (1973) Pathophysiology of acute renal failure. *Arch. Internal Med.*, **131**, 911–928

66. Gömöri, P., Szalay, E. and Zolnay, B. (1965). Corrisive preparations in kidney disease. *Orv. Hetil.,* **106,** 1734. Cited by Renyi-Vamos and Babics (Ref. 154). Some of the corrosion preparations are illustrated by Brod (Ref. 67).
67. Brod, J. (1973). The kidney (London: Butterworths)
68. Matthews, P.G., Morgan, T.O., and Johnston, C.I. (1973). *Nephron,* **10,** 366–367
69. Carriere, S. (1969). Effect of norepinephrine, isoproteronol and adrenergic blockers upon the intrarenal distribution of blood flow. *Can. J. Physiol. Pharmacol.,* **47,** 199–208
70. Dempster, W.J. (1972). The nature of renal perfusion in normal, oliguric and anuric states. *Urologia,* **39,** 2–38
71. Grandchamp, A., Ayer, G. and Truniger, B. (1971). Pathogenesis of redistribution of intrarenal blood flow in haemorrhagic hypotension. *Europ. J. Clin. Invest.,* **1,** 271–276
72. Truniger, B., Rosen, S.M., Grandchamp, A., Strebel, H. and Kriek, H.R. (1971). Redistribution of renal blood flow in hemorrhagic hypotension *Europ. J. Clin. Invest.,* **1,** 277–280
73. Thiel, G., McDonald, F.D., Oken, D.E. (1970). Micropuncture studies of the basis for protection of renin depleted rats from glycerol induced acute renal failure. *Nephron,* **7,** 67–79
74. Chedru, M.F., Baethke, R. and Oken, D.E., (1972). Renal cortical blood flow and glomerular filtration in myohemoglobinuric acute renal failure. *Kidney International,* **1,** 232–239
75. Hutton, I., Pack, A.I., Lindsay, R.M. and Lawrie, T.D.V. (1970). Clinical significance of renal haemodynamics in acute myocardial infarction. *Lancet,* **2,** 123–125
76. Rosenberg, I.K., Gupta, S.L., Lucas, C.E., Khan, A.A. and Rosenberg, B.F. (1971). Renal insufficiency after trauma and sepsis. *Arch. Surg.,* **103,** 178–183
77. Lucas, C.E., Rector, F.E., Wener, M. and Rosenberg, I.K. (1973). Altered renal homeostatis with acute sepsis, *Arch. Surg.,* **106,** 444–449
78. Goormaghtigh, N. (1945). Vascular and circulatory changes in renal cortex in the anuric crush-syndrome. *Proc. Soc. Exp. Biol. Med.,* **59,** 303–305
79. Wilson, D.R., Thiel, G., Arce, M.L. and Oken, D.E. (1969). The role of the concentration mechanism in the development of acute renal failure Micropuncture studies using diabetes insipidus rats. *Nephron,* **6,** 128–139
80. McDonald, F.D., Thiel, G., Wilson, D.R., Dibona, G.F. and Oken, D.E. (1969). The prevention of acute renal failure in the rat by long-term saline loading. *Proc. Soc. Exp. Biol. Med.,* **131,** 610–614
81. Dibona, G.F. and Sawin, L.L. (1971). The renin-angiotensin system in acute renal failure in the rat. *Laboratory Investigation,* **25,** 528–532
82. Fine, L.G. (1970) Acquired prostaglandin in E_2 (medullin) deficiency as the cause of oliguria in acute tubular necrosis. A hypothesis. *Israel J. Med. Sci.,* **6,** 346–350
83. (a): Kokot, F. and Kuska, J. (1969). Plasma renin activity in acute renal insufficiency. *Nephron,* **6,** 115–127
83. (b): Kokot, F. and Kuska, J. (1971). Plasma renin activity in patients with acute and chronic renal insufficiency treated by haemodialysis. *Proc. Europ. Dialysis and Transplant Assn.,* **8,** 542–545

84. Brown, J.J., Gleadle, R.I., Lawson, D.H., Lever, A.F., Linton, A.L., MacAdam, R.F., Prentice, E., Robertson, J.I.S. and Tree, M. (1970). Renin and acute renal failure: Studies in Man. *Brit. Med. J.*, **1**, 253–258
85. Ochoa, E., Finkielman, S. and Agrest, A. (1970). Angiotensin blood levels during the evolution of acute renal failure. *Clin. Sci.*, **38**, 225–231
86. Powell-Jackson, J.D., Brown, J.J., Lever, A.F., MacGregor, J., MacAdam, R.F., Titterington, D.M., Robertson, J.I.S. and Waite, M.A. (1972). Protection against acute renal failure in rats by passive immunisation against angiotensin. *Lancet*, **1**, 774–776
87. *Brit. Med. J.*, (1970). Renin and renal failure. **1**, 250–251
88. Vitsky, B.H., Suzuki, Y., Strauss, L. and Churg, J. (1969). The hemolytic-uremic syndrome. A study of renal pathologic alterations. *Amer. J. Path.*, **57**, 627–647
89. Clarkson, A.R., Lawrence, J.R., Meadows, R. and Seymour, A.E. (1970). The haemolytic uraemic syndrome in adults. *Quart. J. Med.*, **39**, 227–239
90. Robson, J.S., Marin, A.M., Ruckley, V.A. and MacDonald, M.K. (1968). Irreversible post-partum renal failure. *Quart. J. Med.*, **37**, 423–435
91. Clarkson, A.R., Meadows, R. and Lawrence, J.R. (1969). Post-partum renal failure. The generalised Shwartzman reaction. Three further cases and a review. *Australasian Ann. Med.*, **18**, 209–216
92. Churg, J., Koffler, D., Paronetto, F., Rorat, E. and Barnett, R.N. (1970). Hemolytic uremic syndrome as a cause of post-partum renal failure. *Amer. J. Obst. Gynecol.*, **108**, 253–261
93. Ponticelli, C., Imbasciati, E., Tarantino, A., Graziani, G. and Redaelli, B. (1972). Post-partum renal failure with microangiopathic haemolytic anaemia. *Nephron*, **9**, 27–41
94. Brain, M.C. (1970). Microangiopathic hemolytic anemia. *Annual Rev. Med.*, **21**, 133–144
95. Vassali, P. and Richet, G. (1960). Necrose corticale et insufficance renale aiguë des états de choc. *Proc. First International Congress Nephrol.*, 236–302
96. Meyers, B.R., Hirschman, S.Z. and Sloan, W. (1970). Generalized Shwartzman reaction in man after a dog bite. *Ann. Internal Med.*, **73**, 433–438
97. Brun, C. and Munck, O. (1957). Lesions in the kidney in acute renal failure following shock. *Lancet*, **1**, 603–607
98. Olsen, T.S. and Skjoldborg, H. (1967). The fine structure of the renal glomerulus in acute anuria. *Acta Pathologica Microbiologica Scandinavica*, **70**, 205–214
99. Handa, S.P. (1970). Glomerular lesions in acute tubular necrosis. *Postgrad. Med. J.*, **46**, 79–82
100. Sevitt, S. (1956). Distal tubular and proximal tubular necrosis in the kidneys of burned patients. *J. Clin. Path.*, **9**, 279–294
101. Clarkson, A.R., MacDonald, M.K., Fuster, V., Cash, J.D. and Robson, J.S. (1970). Glomerular coagulation in acute ischaemic renal failure. *Quart, J. Med.*, **39**, 585–599
102 Wardle, E.N. and Taylor, G. (1968). Fibrin breakdown products and fibrinolysis in renal disease. *J. Clin. Path.*, **21**, 140–146
103. Haanen, C., Holdrinet, A. and Wijdeveld, P. (1970). Intravascular clotting and acute renal failure. *Scand. J. Haematol.*, **13**, 337–343

104. Larsson, S.O., Hedner, U. and Nilsson, I.M. (1971). On fibrinolytic split products in serum and urine in uraemia. *Scand. J. Urol. Nephr.*, **5**, 234–242
105. Colman, R.W. and Robboy, S.J. and Minna, J.D. (1972). Disseminated intravascular coagulation (DIC): An approach. *Amer. J. Med.*, **52**, 679–689
106. Clarkson, A.R., Sage, R.E. and Lawrence, J.R. (1969). Consumption coagulopathy and acute renal failure due to gram-negative septicemia. after abortion. *Annals Inter. Med.*, **70**, 1191–1199
107. Crisnic, I., Cucuianu, M., Manasia, M. and Uza, G. (1971). Disseminated Intravascular coagulation andacute renal failure. *Thrombosis et Diathesis Haemorrhagica*, **26**, 332–340
108. Kleinknecht, D., Kanfer, A. and Josso, F. (1972). Intravascular coagulation and heparin therapy in acute renal failure: a reappraisal. *Rev. Europ. d'Études Cliniques Biologiques*, **17**, 695–700
109. Weiss, A.E., Easterling, W.E., Odom, M.H., McMillan, C.W., Johnson, A.M. and Talbert, L.M. (1972). Defibrination syndrome after intra-amniotic infusion of hypertonic saline.
113, 868–874
110. Badraqui, M.H.H., Bonnar, J., Hillier, K. and Embrey, M.P. (1973). Coagulation changes during termination of pregnancy by prostaglandins and by vacuum aspiration. *Brit. Med. J.*, **1**, 19–21
111. Preston, F.E., Malia, R.G., Tipton, R.H. and Smith, A.J. (1972). Intravascular coagulation and pre-eclamptic toxaemia. *Lancet*, **1**, 34–35
112. Cornu, P., Soria, J., Soria, C., Morin, P., Strich Mougenot, C., Marsan, C. Laffay, J., Segrestaa, J. -M. and Lamotte, M. (1973). Coagulation intravasculaire disséminée aiguë en milieu obstétrical. *Semaine des Hôpitaux de Paris*, **49**, 1419–1428
113. Pavlou, C. (1973). Disseminated intravascular coagulation with microangiopathic haemolytic anaemia in eclampsia. *Proc. Roy. Soc. Med.*, **66**, 760–761
114. Raby, C., Vairel, E., and Bertrand, H. (1970). Étude de la fonction coagulolytique dans l'insufficance rénale aiguë (IRA). *Presse Medicale*, **78**, 2277–2279
115. Hardaway, R.M. (1966). Syndromes of disseminated intravascular coagulation. With special reference to shock and hemorrhage. (Springfield, Illinois: Charles C. Thomas)
116. Corrigan, J.J. Jr, Ray, W.L. and May, N. (1968). Changes in the blood coagulation system associated with septicemia. *New Eng. J. Med.*, **279**, 851–856
117. Harker, L.A. and Slichter, S.S. (1972). Platelet and fibrinogen consumption in man. *New Eng. J. Med.*, **287**, 999–1005
118. Wardle, E.N. (1972). Intravascular coagulation in infection: A study by radio-fibrinogen. *Scand. J. Infectious Diseases*, **4**, 155–159
119. Preston., F.E., Malia, R.G., Sworn, M.J. and Blackburn, E.K. (1973). Intravascular coagualtion and *E. Coli* septicaemia. *J. Clin. Path.* **26**, 120–125
120. Jaroonvesama, N. (1972). Intravascular coagulation in falciparum malaria. *Lancet.*, **1**, 221–223
121. Reid, H.A. and Nkrumah, F.K. (1972). Fibrin-degradation products in cerebral malaria. *Lancet*, **1**, 218–221
122. Vachon, F., Carbon, C., Beaufils, P. and Vic-Dupont, V. (1973). L'insufficance rénale aiguë du paludisme pernicieux. *La Nouv. Press Med.*, **2**, 1035–1039

123. Simon, G.T. and Giacobino, J.P. (1970). Pathogenisis of the glomerular lesions in acute pancreatitis. *Lancet,* **2,** 669–670
124. Axton, J.H.M. (1972). Six cases of poisoning after a parenteral organic mercurial compound (Merthiolate). *Postgrad. Med. J.* **48,** 417–421
125. Weiss, H.J., Berger, R.E., Tice, A.D., Philips, L.L. (1972). Fatal disseminated intravascular coagulation and hemolytic anemia following stibophen therapy. *Amer. J. Med. Sc.,* **264,** 375–384
126. Menon, I.S., Dewar, H.A. and Newell, D.J. (1968). Role of the kidney in fibrinolytic activity of blood, *Lancet,* **1,** 785–788
127. Humair, L. Potter, E.V. and Kwaan, H.C. (1969). The role of fibrinogen in renal disease. *J. Lab. Clin. Med.,* **74,** 60–71
128. Diethelm, A.G. and Wilson, S.J. (1971). Obstruction to the renal microcirculation after temporary ischemia. *J. Surg. Res.,* **11,** 265–276
129. Wardle, E.N. (1973a). Acute renal failure following injection of procoagulants. Submitted to *J. Lab. Clin. Med.*
130. Skjørten, F. (1969). Hyaline microthrombi in an autopsy material. *Acta Path. Microbiol. Scand.,* **76,** 361–375
131. Wardle, E.N. (1973b). Fibrin in renal disease: functional considerations. Submitted to *Clin. Nephrology*
132. Wardle, E.N. (1973c). Fibrinogen catabolism studies in patients with renal disease. *Quart. J. Med.,* **52,** 205
133. Luke, R.G., Briggs, J.D., Allison, M.E.M. and Kennedy, A.C. (1970). Factors determining response to mannitol in acute renal failure. *Amer. J. Med. Sci.,* **259,** 168–174
134. Peters, J.T. (1945). Oliguria and anuria due to increased intrarenal pressure. *Annal. Internal Med.,* **23,** 221–236
135. Abeshouse, B.S. (1945). Renal decapsulation: A review of the literature and a report of ten cases. *J. Urol.,* **53,** 27–84
136. De Wardener, H.E. (1955). Intrarenal pressure in experimental tubular necrosis. *Lancet,* **1,** 580–584
137. Brun, C., Crone, C., Davidsen, H.G., Fabricus, J., Hansen, A.T., Lassen, N.A. and Munck, O. (1956). Renal interstitial pressure in normal and in anuric man: based on wedged renal vein pressure. *Proc. Soc. Exp. Biol. Med.,* **91,** 199–202
138. Sims, E.A.H., Goldberg, H.I., Kelly, J.R. and Sisco, B. (1959). Glomerular perfusion during acute renal insufficiency from mercury poisoning in the rat. *J. Lab. Clin. Med.,* **54,** 440–449
139. Bank, N., Mutz, B.F. and Aynedjian, H.S. (1967). The role of 'leakage' of tubular fluid in anuria due to mercury poisoning. *J. Clin. Invest.,* **46,** 695–704
140. Barenberg, R.L., Solomon, S., Papper, S. and Anderson, R. (1968). Clearance and micropuncture study of renal function in mercuric chloride treated rats. *J. Lab. Clin. Med.,* **72,** 473–483
141. Lucke, B. (1946). Lower nephron nephrosis (renal lesions of the crush syndrome of burns, transfusions, and other conditions affecting lower segment of nephrons. *Military surgeon,* **99,** 371–396
142. Sevitt, S. (1959). Pathogenisis of traumatic uremia; a revised concept. *Lancet,* **2,** 135–141
143. Meroney, W.H. and Rubini, M.E. (1959). Kidney function during acute tubular necrosis. *Metabolism,* **8,** 1–15
144. Finckh, E.S. Jeremy, D. and Whyte, H.M. (1962). Structural renal damage and its relation to clinical features in acute oliguric renal failure *Quart. J. Med.,* **31,** 429–446

145. Olsen, T.S. (1967). Ultrastructure of the renal tubules in acute renal insufficiency. *Acta Path. Microbiol. Scand.*, **71**, 203–218
146. Henry, L.N., Lane, C.E. and Kashgarian, M. (1968). Micropuncture studies of the pathophysiology of acute renal failure in the rat. *Lab. Invest.*, **19**, 309–314
147. Brenner, B.M., Troy, J.L., Daugharty, T.M. (1971). The dynamics of glomerular ultrafiltration in the rat. *J. Clin. Invest.* **50**, 1776–1780
148. Walker, J.G., Silva, H., Lawson, T.R., Ryder, J.A. and Shaldon, S. (1963). Renal blood flow in acute renal failure measured by renal arterial infusion of indocyanine green. *Proc. Soc. Exp. Biol. Med. (New York)*, **112**, 932–935
149. Munck, O. (1964). Renal circulation in acute renal failure measured with radioactive krypton-85 and xenon-133. *A Symposium*. Ed. by S. Shaldon and G.C. Cook, (Oxford: Blackwell)
150. Reubi, F.C., Gossweiler, N. and Gurtler, R. (1966). Renal circulation in man studied by means of dye-dilution method. *Circulation*, **33**, 426–442
151. Shaldon, S., Sheville, E. and Rae, A.I. (1964). Angiography in acute renal failure. *Clin. Radiol.*, **15**, 123–129
152. Hollenberg, N.K., Sandor, T., Conroy, M., Adams, D.F., Solomon, H.S., Abrams, H.L. and Merrill, J.P. (1973). Xenon transit through the oliguric human kidney; Analysis by maximum likelihood. *Kidney International*, **3**, 177–185
153. Suzuki, T. and Mostofi, F.K. (1970). Electron microscopic studies of acute tubular necrosis. Early changes in the glomeruli of the rat kidney after subcutaneous injection of glycerin. *Lab. Invest.*, **23**, 8–14
154. Renyi-Vamos, F. and Babics, A. (1972). Anuria. Therapeutic experiences. (London: Pitman Medical)
155. Pasternack, A., Tallqvist, G. and Kuhlback, B. (1970). Occurrence of interstitial nephritis in acute renal failure. *Acta Med. Scand.*, **187**, 27–31
156. Di Bona, G.F., McDonald, F.D., Flamembaum, W., Dammin, G.F. and Oken, D.E. (1971). Maintenance of renal function in salt loaded rats despite severe tubular necrosis induced by HgC_2. *Nephron*, **8**, 205–220
157. Darmady, E.M. and Stranack, F. (1955). Microdissection of renal tubules. *Proc. Roy. Soc. Med.*, **48**, 781–783
158. Thiel, G., Wilson, D.R., Arce, M.L. and Oken, D.E. (1967). Glycerol induced hemoglobinuric acute renal failure in the rat. 2. The experimental model, predisposing factors and pathophysiologic features. *Nephron*, **4**, 276–297
159. Elliott, R.W. and Kerr, D.N.S. (1967). Post-operative renal failure. *Newcastle Med. J.*, **29**, 290–298

Chapter 3

RADIOLOGY IN ACUTE RENAL FAILURE

T. Sherwood

There was very little radiology of acute renal failure (ARF) to discuss until about 10 years ago. The intravenous urogram (IVU) was thought to be useless and dangerous in all renal failure states, and plain films of the chest, abdomen and hands, together with occasional arteriograms, made up the repertoire of radiological investigation. Nephrologists will not need reminding that since then the IVU has grown into a most rewarding investigation in ARF. For the successful renal failure IVU, it is essential to avoid preliminary dehydration, to recognise that a careful radiographic technique using tomograms is critical, and to give an adequate dose of the contrast medium[1]. In the great majority of patients with renal failure, it is then possible to achieve a nephrogram – a diffuse opacification of the kidneys. The important questions to be asked of the IVU in this state are quite limited[2], with the nephrogram often of decisive help. In any patient with ARF we need to know: (i) where and how large are the kidneys; (ii) can obstruction be excluded with confidence: and (iii) are there any clues as to aetiology?

Renal size and site are of obvious importance to the diagnosis of acute, as opposed to acute-on-chronic, renal failure, and to successful renal biopsy.

As an unusual but treatable cause of ARF, *urinary tract obstruction* is a vital matter for consideration in all patients. In the past retrograde pyelography has always been thought essential to avoid tragic diagnostic failures here. To this end there should certainly never be any hesitation in carrying out this investigation in the doubtful case. However, the IVU can now help to cut down the need for retrograde studies to a minimum. In long-standing obstructive states the nephrogram has a characteristic appearance: the dilated non-opacified calices present as lucent, regular, spherical defects against the opacified renal parenchyma.

Whilst this picture is diagnostic, its absence must never be taken to exclude obstruction. The importance of routine delayed films, up to at least 24 hours after contrast medium injection, can hardly be overstressed for the confident IVU exclusion of obstruction. These late films will show a typical pyelogram in obstruction, with dilated renal pelvis and ureters, provided enough contrast medium has entered the nephrons to produce a nephrogram on the earlier films. We have sometimes come uncomfortably close to missing the diagnosis only in those patients in whom we failed to carry out late films. With care, the IVU can thus exclude urinary tract obstruction, i.e. in the presence of an even dense nephrogram that does not advance to an obstructive pyelogram 24 hours later. In those few patients with ARF who do not show a nephrogram during the IVU, a severe perfusion or filtration defect is likely, but obstruction cannot be excluded.

Distinctive Nephrogram Patterns in Man

It is occasionally possible to reach a final diagnosis in ARF on the IVU alone, e.g. when a characteristic patchy nephrogram outlines large uneven kidneys: acute-on-chronic failure in polycystic disease. The IVU finding of central interest in the oliguric patient, however, is the dense even nephrogram.

The occurrence of an immediate, dense, long-lasting nephrogram is wholly characteristic of ARF linked with the histological diagnosis of *acute tubular necrosis* (ARF/ATN). In severe oliguria this is, at first sight, a surprising finding, and clearly demands a close understanding of the handling of contrast medium by the kidney. There is now a considerable body of evidence that glomerular filtration is the only important route of excretion for the current urographic contrast media, with no tubular excretion or re-absorption. The IVU is therefore an upper nephron event, determined by glomerular filtration rate, the plasma level of contrast medium, and proximal tubular water re-absorption[3]. Its occurrence in ARF/ATN must imply a measure of continuing glomerular filtration in this state[4].

Fry and Cattell[5] have suggested a useful framework for studying abnormal nephrogram patterns in human disease. Leaving aside the faint long-lasting nephrogram met in severe glomerular disease, as in chronic glomerulo-nephritis, they divide the abnormal dense nephrogram into two patterns. They contrast the immediate persistent nephrogram of ARF/ATN, also seen in acute suppurative pyelonephritis, with a pattern where the nephrogram may begin feebly, but grows increasingly dense over the minutes and hours of the investigation. This second pattern is the familiar one of *acute extra-renal obstruction* by a ureteric calculus, and also occurs in *renal hypotensive and ischaemic states.* In these three disorders there is good evidence pointing to continuing glomerular filtration by displacement, i.e. water movement into and out of the nephron by filtration and tubular water re-absorption. This provides a ready vehicle for carrying contrast medium into the nephron where it accumulates, accounting for the increasingly dense nephrogram. A particularly interesting example of this pattern occurs in the *medullary necrosis* of infancy, where it may also present as a more localised abnormal density outlining necrotic papillae[6]

If the ARF/ATN nephrogram appears at once and does not grow denser over the hours and days that it may last, contrast medium carried into the nephron by glomerular filtration might be supposed to be re-absorbed across the damaged tubular cell, back into the circulation. This is certainly a possibility, supported by recent work on the constancy of this nephrogram pattern in ARF/ATN[7]. In a preliminary study of patients at Hammersmith and St. Peter's Hospitals, we have found that nephrograms may occasionally cross boundaries, so that out of 30 patients with ARF/ATN, a third appeared to show nephrograms that did increase in density with time (Figure 3.1). This in no way invalidates a very useful clinical nephrogram framework, but may make the need for finding mechanisms of the contrast medium leaving the kidney rather less pressing (Sherwood *et al.*, unpublished observations).

The functional basis of the abnormal ARF/ATN nephrogram is a fascinating problem, and must involve discussion of experimental observations on the disturbed renal haemodynamic state in this disorder.

Experimental ARF – Renal Vascular Shut-down

The observation that the kidney may respond to various insults by selective outer cortical ischaemia[8] was soon confused by dissent over an intra-renal shunt proposed in this work. However, cortical vascular shut-down, e.g. during haemorrhagic hypotension in the dog, can be clearly shown by current, fine detail angiographic methods[9]. This is not simply the non-specific response of the

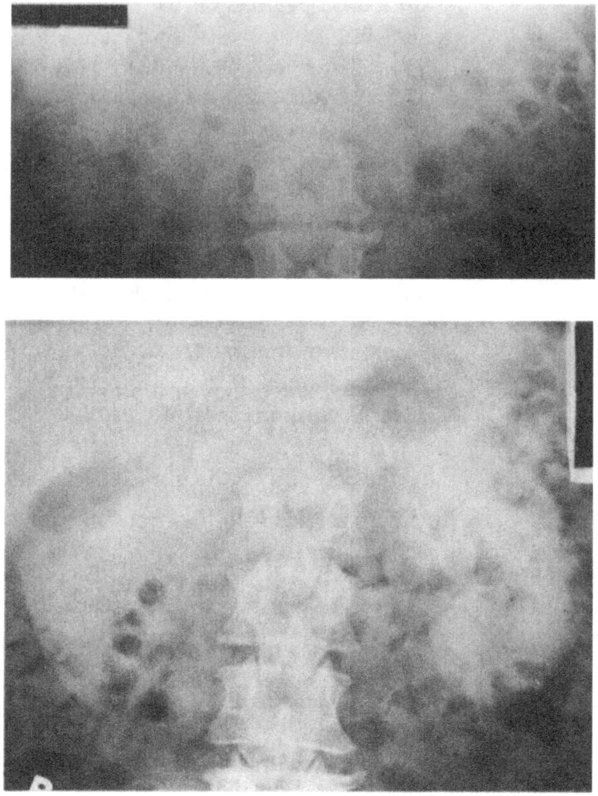

Figure 3.1 (a) Intravenous urogram in a patient with ARF/ATN following a severe crush injury. Above: control film – the kidneys cannot be seen Below: 10 min after contrast medium injection – there is an obvious bilateral nephrogram.

renal cortex to a falling renal blood flow: it is possible to show by means of aortic balloon experiments that the cortical vascular bed remains widely open at very low perfusion pressure and flow[10].

The view that renal vascular shut-down is a common and important event in ARF/ATN rests on angiographic, gas radioisotope, labelled microsphere, and micropuncture evidence, and has been summarised by Earley[11] and Oken[12]. Of the possible mechanisms leading to renal cortical ischaemia, angiography can be used for excluding some obvious extra-renal candidates, e.g. catechol

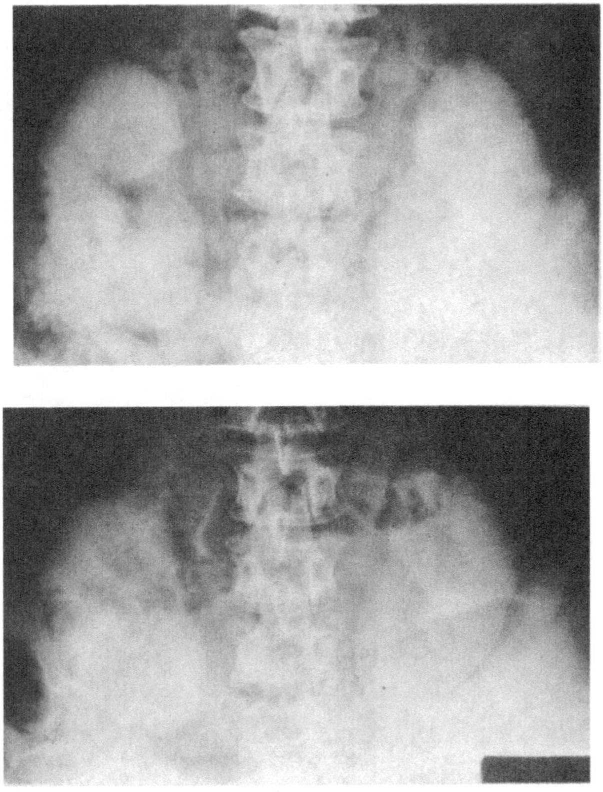

Figure 3.1 (b). 5 hours (above) and 18 hours (below) later, the density of the nephrogram is still increasing. The patient's renal biopsy findings and his complete recovery supported the diagnosis.

amines and renal innervation[13]. Professor Kerr has already discussed possible intra-renal mechanisms, among them the renin–angiotensin system[14], and no one following him would wish to try bludgeoning you with yet another unitary explanation for ARF/ATN.

It is perhaps helpful to attempt moving away from the concept of active vasoconstriction inevitably associated with vascular shut-down notions. A much more mechanical basis for these events can be investigated. Elegant experiments on the ischaemic brain and kidney have shown that a 'no-reflow phenomenon'

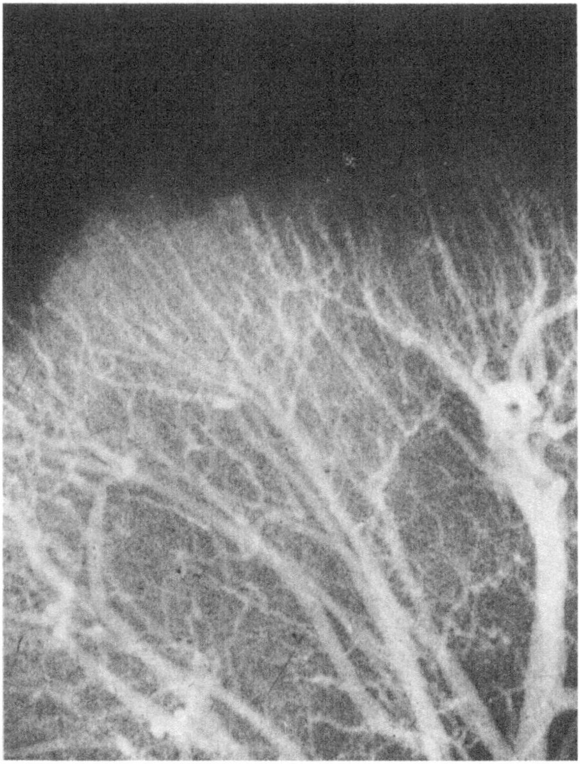

Figure 3.2 *In vivo* renal arteriogram in the dog following intravenous mercuric chloride (0.5 mg/kg). There is severe cortical shut-down: the tree-in-winter appearance, with branches of main vessels standing out starkly in the absence of glomerular background filling. Renal blood flow measured by electromagnetic flow probe has also fallen sharply.

occurs on restoring the circulation, very probably related to red cell trapping by capillary channels narrowed to a critical diameter[15,16] Cell volume is the important consideration here, with osmotic swelling of the sick cell, no longer able to extrude sodium.

We have been interested that the ARF/ATN stated induced in the dog by intravascular mercury follows these ideas closely. We have found an immediate fall in renal blood flow, together with characteristic cortical shut-down on angiography, when a small amount of mercuric chloride is introduced into the circulation in these animals (Figure 3.2). This effect is not mediated by glomerular filtration, as it also occurs in the kidney deprived of filtration pressure. It is of particular interest that in the same animal, one kidney can be thrown into shut-down by a small renal artery mercury bolus, and the contralateral kidney completely protected from similar shut down by hyperosmolar mannitol (Figure 3.3). Such observations are in accord with a toxic, 'swollen cell' capillary block as the basis of cortical ischaemia in nephrotoxin induced ARF/ATN (Sherwood *et al.*, unpublished observations).

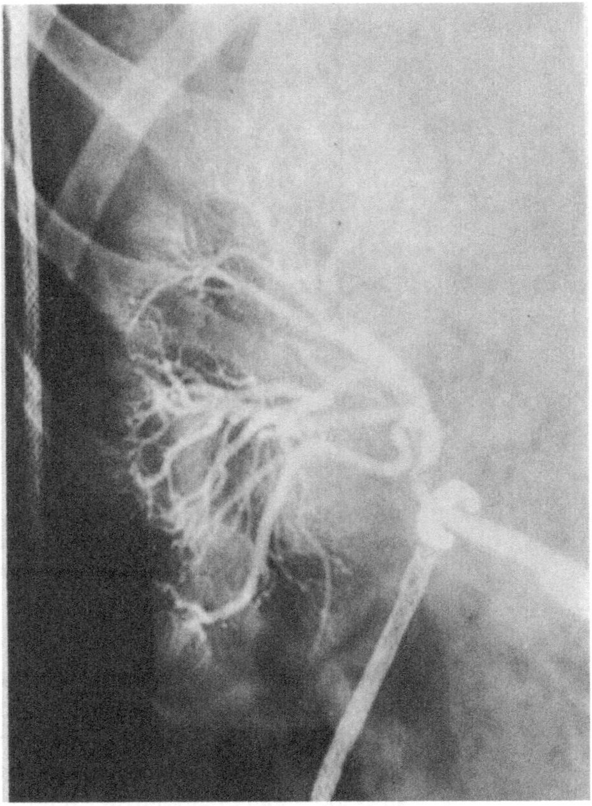

Figure 3.3 (a) ***In vivo*** **renal arteriogram in the dog following a mercuric chloride (5 mg) bolus into the right renal artery: a severe fall in renal blood flow is matched by the picture of extensive, patchy cortical shut-down.**

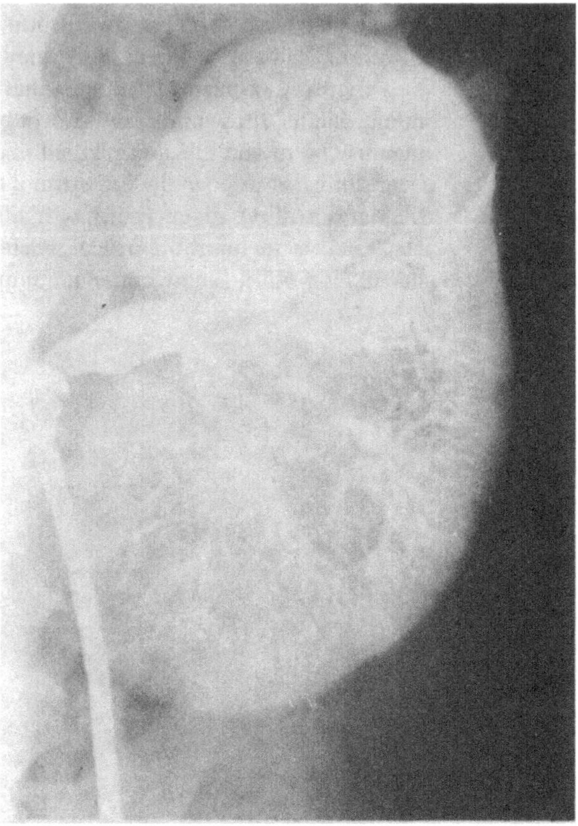

Figure 3.3 (b) Following a systemic infusion of hyperosmolar mannitol, a similar mercury bolus has now been injected into the left renal artery. There is no fall in renal blood flow, and the renal arteriogram shows a normal vascular bed.

Conclusion

If outer cortical ischaemia is the dominant event in ARF/ATN, then the immediate dense nephrogram characteristic of the IVU in this state has an almost too ready explanation[17]. Outer cortical nephrons have a different structure and function, with their short loops and predominant excretory service, to inner cortical units with their long loops geared to re-absorption and concentration. Shut-down of the outer cortex is thus associated with oliguria, but continuing filtration in inner cortical glomeruli. With nephrogram mechanics so dependent on filtration and water reabsorption, this is an attractive notion.

Clearly there is now a radiology of ARF. Interesting uncertainty may remain on basic mechanisms, but there is little doubt that sound clinical help can be expected from the renal failure IVU. The immediate dense nephrogram of ARF/ATN is among the most rewarding of findings, pointing to a recoverable renal lesion.

References

1. Fry, I.K. and Cattell, W.R. (1971). Radiology in the diagnosis of renal failure. *Brit. Med. Bull.,* **27,** 148–152
2. Schwartz, W.B., Hurwit, A. and Ettinger, A. (1963). Intravenous urography in the patient with renal insufficiency. *New Eng. J. Me.,* **269,** 277–283
3. Sherwood, T. (1971). The physiology of intravenous urography. *Scientific Basis of Medicine Annual Reviews,* Chap. 19, (London: Athlone Press)
4. Chamberlain, M.J. and Sherwood, T. (1967). Intravenous urography in experimental acute renal failure in the rat. *Nephron,* **4,** 65–74
5. Chrispin, A.R. (1972). Medullary necrosis in infancy. *Brit. Med. Bull.,* **28,** 233–236
6. Cattell, W.R., McIntosh, C.S., Moseley, I.F. and Fry, I.K. (1973). Excretion urography in acute renal failure. *Brit. Med. J.,* **2,** 575–578
7. Trueta, J., Barclay, A.E., Daniel, P.M., Franklin, K.J. and Prichard, M.M. L., (1947). Studies of the renal circulation. (Oxford: Blackwell Scientific Publications).
8. Lavender, J.P., Sherwood, T. and Russelll, S. (1969). *In vivo* renal microangiography. *Brit. J. Radio.,* **42,** 247–251
9. Lavender, J.P. and Sherwood, T. (1971). The renal cortex angiogram and renal blood flow. *Brit. J. Radio.,* **44,** 505–510
10. Earley, L.E. (1970). Pathogensis of oliguric acute renal failure. *New Eng. J. Med.,* **282,** 1370–1371
11. Oken, D.E. (1971). Nosologic considerations in the nomenclature of acute renal failure. *Nephron,* **8,** 505–510
12. Lavender, J.P. and Sherwood, T. (1972). The renal circulation in haemorrhagic hypotension. *Brit. Med. Bull.,* **28,** 241–246
13. Brown, J.J., Gleadle, R.I., Lawson, D.H., Lever, A.F., Linton, A.L., Macadam, R.F., Prentice, E., Robertson, J.I.S. and Tree, M. (1970). Renin and acute renal failure. *Brit. Med. J.,* **1,** 253–258
14. Flores, J., Di Bona, D.R., Beck, C.H. and Leaf, A. (1972). The role of cell swelling in ischaemic renal damage and the protective effect of hypertonic solute. *J. Clin. Invest.,* **51,** 118–126
15. Leaf, A. (1970). Regulation of intracellular fluid volume and disease. *Amer. J. Med.,* **49,** 291–295
16. Dempster, W.J. (1971). The nature of experimental second-set kidney transplant rejection 5. *Brit. J. Ex. Path.,* **52,** 594–609
17. Fry, I.K. and Cattell, W.R. (1972). The nephrographic pattern during excretion urography. *Brit. Med. Bull.,* **28,** 227–232

Chapter 4

THE RENAL LESION IN ACUTE TUBULOINTERSTITIAL NEPHROPATHY
(Alias "Acute Tubular Necrosis")

C. Brun

Since shortly after the rediscovery of post-traumatic acute renal failure during World War 2 it has been assumed that renal ischaemia and hypoxia is the causative mechanism of this potentially reversible renal condition, and that the typical histological lesion is tubular necrosis. Acute tubular necrosis is the name at which the roulette has stopped at present – even if this name, in my opinion, is largely undeserved. During the long and rather curious life history of this nephrological entity, many different and more or less meaningful names have been used – most of which I will omit. The life history is curious because this disease, which was known decades before World War 1, tended to drop out of the medical spectrum between the natural or man-made catastrophes which gave rise to new crops of cases. During World War 2 it was known to the Germans, who named it vasomotorische nephrosis and separated it from the, at that time prevalent, trench nephritis, and a number of German papers including some doctoral theses were written on this subject[1-4]. On the Allied side it seems to have been unknown and the very comprehensive publications by the Medical Research Committee on *'Surgical Shock and Allied Conditions'* [5] does not mention renal failure following shock. Between the two world wars the disease was forgotten and rediscovered at least twice[6,7], and each time presented as a new entity. When World War 2 produced considerable numbers of cases, the medical world was again surprised to see acute renal failure develop following traumatic shock, crush injuries, etc. In Britain many cases were seen during the heavy bombardments of London in the winter of 1940–1941 and a number of papers were published in the *British Medical Journal* in 1941. The histological changes described included tubular dilation, formation of pigmented casts and tubular damage, including necrosis. The latter changes are in the first paper[8] peculiarly enough stated to have been located in the proximal tubules while in later papers they seem to have been moved to the distal convoluted tubules without further ado.

After the War Lucke published a vast number of cases from U.S. Army Institute of Pathology and coined the term 'Lower Nephron Nephrosis'[9]. His main findings were: (i) Focal degeneration of necrosis in the epithelium of the ascending limb of Henle's loop and the distal convoluted tubule. (ii) Interstitial oedema and cellular infiltration. (iii) Pigmented casts in the distal parts of the nephron. (iv) Few or no changes in the glomeruli, the proximal tubules and the descending limb of Henle's loop.

The term acute tubular necrosis seems to have been introduced in 1950 in an important paper 'Renal Function Studies in Acute Tubular Necrosis' by Bull, Joekes and Lowe[10]. Many papers on the disease have since appeared in a steady flow and the risk that it should again fall into oblivion is now remote – the accidents on our roads and the complications connected with heroic surgery will see to that, even if the numbers of post-abortion cases might diminish or nearly disappear. All the early and most of the later papers are based on studies of post mortem material and it is obvious that due to autolytic changes studies of degenerative changes and even of frank necrosis in the tubular epitherlium is at best very difficult – and in many cases quite impossible. With the introduction of percutaneous renal biopsy in 1949[11] it became possible to study renal tissue without autolyte changes and also to study less severe non-fatal cases, and to do repeat biopsies. Tissue for electron-microscopic studies could also be obtained. One of the first clinical problems to which the new biopsy method was turned was acute renal failure[12].

Biopsy Studies

The most striking light microscopical observation in biopsies from even severe cases of acute renal failure of the type under discussion here (I avoid deliberately using the name 'tubular necrosis'), is the paucity of changes. The few histological changes found are quite out of proportion to the very severe reduction in, or even complete abolition of, renal function seen in these cases. Tubular necrosis is rare if even seen at all, and definitely not the typical lesion to look for in a biopsy from a patient with acute renal failure[13]. The following is a summary of the lesions as seen by light microscopy in our biopsy material which has been collected over more than 20 years. It is classified as acute tubulo-interstitial nephropathy (a.t.i.n.).

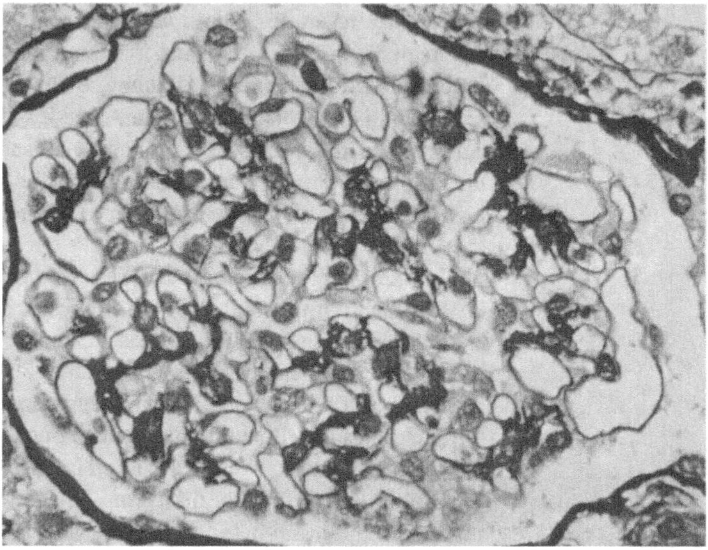

Figure 4.1 Acute Renal Failure. Glomerulus with patient capillaries, no hypercellularity and normal basement membranes. The Bowmans Capsule is likewise normal. 2 µm section, silvermethenamine + H & E, original magnification 520X .

Bowmans Capsule Normal. Intrusion of proximal epithelium in the capsule has been described, but this can be seen also in normals.

Glomeruli Normal. Occasionally an increase in the number of granulocytes can be seen – especially if the patient has leukocytosis. The number of erythrocytes seen in the capillary tuft is normal.

Proximal Tubules Often normal. If the patient has been given mannitol or dextran infusion, so called 'hydropic change' can be seen in the epithelium, which contains numerous clear vacuoles. The nuclei are normal and necrosis is never seen. Casts are absent.

Distal Tubules (Including the ascending limb of Henle's loop): These are focally dilated and lined with a flattened epithelium. The cross-sections are often of a 'pretzel' like configuration. Pigmented casts are nearly always found, but to a varying degree. The casts are mostly granular, often containing visible residues of degraded erythrocytes Occasionally focal necrosis of a single tubule or some of its epithelial cells is found, but extensive tubular necrosis is not seen. The necroses, if present, are mainly found where a cast is located. The tubulovenous anastomoses described in the early papers have not been found in renal biopsies in our series.

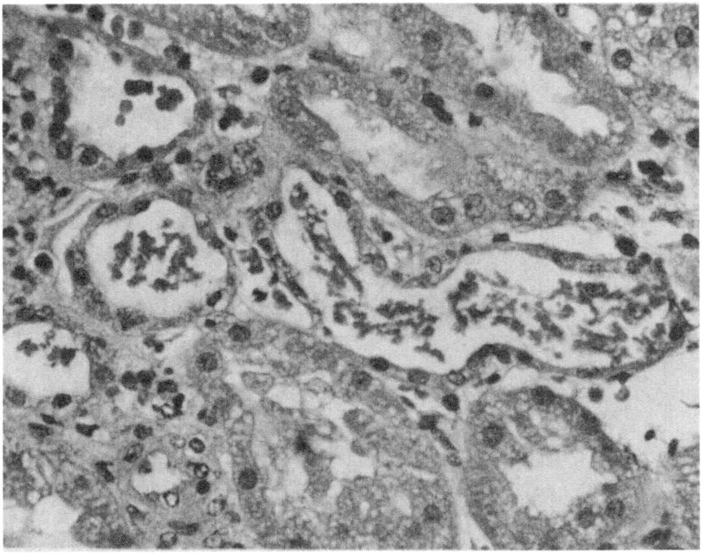

Figure 4.2 Dilated distal tubules lined with flattened, but not necrotic epithelium, containing pigmented granular masses. 4 μm section, H & E, original magnification 325X.

Vessels Normal

Interstitial Tissue Slight to moderate focal oedema and focal cellular infiltration of lymphocytes, plasma cells and granulocytes in varying proportions and degrees is nearly always observed. The interstitial oedema

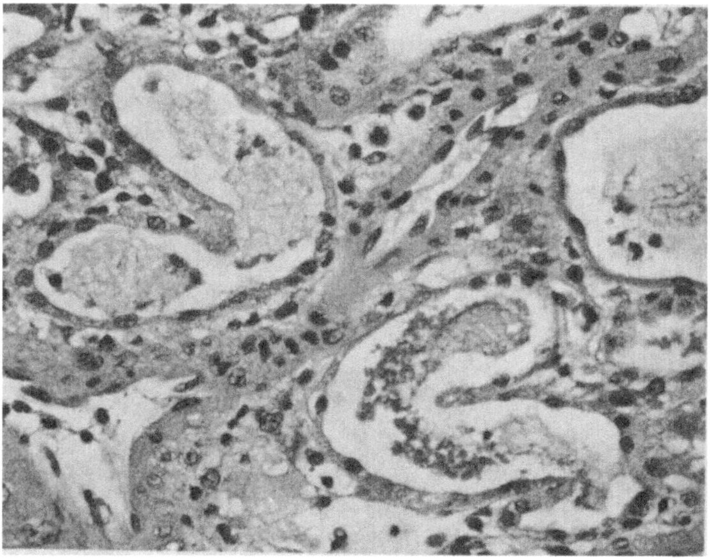

Figure 4.3 As Figure 4.2. Note the typical pretzel-like configuration.

can be generalised and pronounced in overhydrated patients. Extratubular masses of brownish material can occasionally be found in the interstitium, presumably a cast extruded from a tubule.

Table 4.1 Light Microscopy

Normal glomeruli
Normal or slightly dilated proximal tubules
Dilated distal tubules lined w. flattened epithelium
'Pretzel-like' cross-sections
Pigmented casts in the distal tubules, loop of Henle and collecting ducts
Patchy interstitial oedema and cellular infiltration
Little or no tubular necrosis

Electron Microscopic Studies

Steen Olsen[14,15] studied twelve biopsies from ten patients with the clinical picture of typical acute renal failure following surgical or obstetrical complications, extensive wounds, sulphonamide reaction or barbiturate poisoning. These biopsies were compared with four controls from patients with normal renal function. Glomeruli were invariably found to be normal and the proximal tubules were either normal or contained single membrane-bounded vacuolar structures in the cytoplasm if the patients had received mannitol or dextran. Cells with what could be called 'osmotic' vacuoles contained normally-structured mitochondria and nuclei. The distal tubules were distended, lined with flat cells and contained casts in which fragments of epithelial cells, possibly haemoglobin, and fibrin-like material could be identified. The epithelial cells showed moderate changes of ultra-structural detail. Unquestionable necroses were seen only in one biopsy. Characteristically, the few necrotic cells observed were bordered by preserved non-necrotic cells. Clarkson *et al.*[16] in an electron microscopical study found occlusive intracapillary fibrin deposition and thrombus formation in the capillaries of glomeruli which were normal by light microscopy. In a later paper[17] from the same group it is stated that by electron microscopy one may over-assess the degree of fibrin deposition and that immunofluorescence microscopy is a better technique for fibrin detection. No glomerular coagulation could be found in Olsen's cases.

Table 4.2 Electron microscopy

Glomeruli:	No significant changes
Proximal tubules:	Insignificant changes or vacuolisation (following administration of dextran, Mannitol etc.)
Distal tubules:	Dilation. Flattening of epithelium. Casts (haemoglobin, fibrin, cytoplasmic debris) Little or no tubular necrosis (patchy if present)

Discussion

What then is the cause of the discrepancy between the changes seen in biopsies by light and electron microscopy and what might be called the 'classical' descriptions? One immediate explanation is that when the term acute tubular necrosis was coined all renal tissue which was available for study was post mortem material. It is literally impossible to attempt investigations which includes a detailed study of the tubular epithelia in post mortem material because autolytic changes in these cells sets in very rapidly after death and cannot be differentiated from *in vivo* degenerative changes. That the 'military' cases seen during wars should be of a different and even more severe type than the civilian cases today is not likely.

I am tempted to believe that over-emphasis has been placed on the presence of tubular necrosis in the early descriptions of the histological changes, and that this idea has been perpetuated without too much speculation even after biopsy material and ultrastructural studies were available.

The name acute tubular necrosis is thus an inappropriate designation which is not better than Lucké's term lower nephron nephrosis and less truly descriptive than acute tubulo-interstitial nephropathy. However, tubular necrosis has at least in many places served the communication between pathologist and clinician tolerably well for years. Our medical terminology is full of nonsensical names and sloppy definitions (e.g. nephrosis, nephrotic syndrome and amyloidosis) and one should possibly not bother too much to change names as long as they are not directly misleading. But this is exactly what is happening to tubular necrosis. The nephropathologist working with tissue from renal grafts unavoidably and quite frequently meets true tubular necrosis caused by thrombus formation in the larger arteries of the graft, or by too long a period of warm ischaemia. These changes cannot be diagnosed as 'acute tubular necrosis' since the words are already in use for the reversible type of acute renal failure which I have just described as tubulo-interstitial nephropathy. This latter entity is an important differential diagnosis in renal graft pathology and must necessarily be separated from vascular rejection and from thrombotic events for obvious therapeutic reasons.

Conclusion

Studies of renal biopsies from patients with post-traumatic acute renal failure have shown characteristic histological changes which are easily recognisable by light microscopy, but which only rarely includes tubular necrosis. To avoid confusion of terminology – especially in renal graft pathology – it is suggested that the designation acute tubular necrosis is replaced by acute tubulo-interstitial nephropathy.

References

1. Borst, M. (1917). *Sammlung Klinische Vorträge (Volkmann)*, **735**, 328
2. Hackradt, A. (1917). *Inaugural-Dissertation*, München
3. Lewin, A. (1919). *Inaugural-Dissertation*, Berlin
4. Bredauer, K. (1920). *Inaugural-Dissertation*, München
5. Research Council Report Series (1919). *Reports of the Special Investigation Committee on Surgical Shock and Allied Conditions*, **25**, 1 and **26**, 8 (London)
6. Husfeldt, E. and Bjering, T. (1937). *Acta Med. Scand.*, **91**, 279
7. Kimmelstiel, P. (1938). *Amer. J. Path.*, **14**, 737
8. Bywaters, E.G.L. and Beall, D. (1941). *Brit. Med. J.*, **1**, 427
9. Lucké, B (1946). *Mil. Surg.*, **99**, 371
10. Bull, G.M., Joekes, A.M. and Lowe, K.G. (1950). *Clin. Science*, **9**, 379
11. Iversen, P. and Brun, C. (1951). *Amer. J. Med.*, **11**, 324
12. Brun, C., *Acute Anuria*, Thesis 1954, (Copenhagen: Munksgaard)
13. Brun, C. and Munck, O. (1957). *Lancet*, **1**, 603
14. Olsen, Steen T. and Skjoldborg, (1967). *Acta Path. Microbiol. Scand.*, **70**, 205
15. Olsen, Steen, T. (1967). *Acta Path. Microbiol. Scand.*, **71**, 203
16. Clarkson, A.R., MacDonald, Mary K., Furster, V., Cash, J.D. and Robson, J.S. (1970). *Quart. J. Med.*, **156**, 585
17. Davidson, A.M., Thomson, D., MacDonald, Mary K., Rae, J.K., Uttley, W.S. and Clarkson, A.R. (1973). *J. Clin. Path.*, **26**, 102

Discussion – First Session

Jackson (Royal Air Force) *I would like to ask Dr Kerr about renal failure and muscle necrosis. I have personally seen eight patients who have had proven muscle necrosis after exercise. Some Americans, in their exercises, do squat jumps down on their quadriceps and many of them get dark urine; they pass quite a lot of myoglobin and of course many of these go into mild or sometimes severe renal failure. It seems very odd that these people should do this when there is so much exercise performed in the world and only these few come out with serious damage.*

Professor Kerr (Newcastle) *I think quite a proportion of the American cases have occurred in people who were also suffering from heat exhaustion, in whom presumably there was a predisposition to renal damage by reduced* **extra-cellular** *fluid volume and renal vaso-constriction, but I think there is little doubt that in some of the patients you are describing it is reasonable to assume that the release of some substance of muscle is responsible. You have these patients with idiopathic rhabdomyolysis who produce the same syndrome, again without any obvious evidence of shock, but although I provocatively put forward the suggestion that it is all due to myoglobin casts in the tubules one cannot really scientifically put that suggestion forward. The fact that an occasional one gets a diuresis with diuretics proves really nothing and I think it is purely on the grounds of probability one suggests this is the mechanism.*

Jackson *Just to mention some of the cases. One was a Dutch soldier taking part in the Niejmegen march on a very hot day, and two others were associated with this and of course there was one in Tripoli during forced marching, so there probably is an agravating factor.*

Dr Dunnill (Oxford) *I would like to ask Dr Kerr about the pathogenesis of the oliguria. He poured great scorn on the theory of back filtration and yet Dr Sherwood shows that in this condition of acute renal failure the nephrogram depends on the presence of a glomerular filtrate and yet you get an increased density of the nephrogram days even after the original injury and this surely points to the fact that glomerular filtration is going on.*

Kerr *I would not say that I scorned the suggestion of back filtration. I dismissed it quickly, among many suggestions, purely on the grounds that in animal models of acute tubular necrosis (which notoriously are not exactly the same as the human disease) glomerular filtration seems to have ceased. As to why you get oliguria, I think this has been shown by at least anecdotal evidence to be related to the degree of depression of the GFR. Patients with non-oliguric acute renal failure have a few ml per-minute of GFR left and the disease is largely diagnosed in situations like burns and head injuries where the patients are having their renal function monitored from the word go. So I think my impression is that oliguric acute renal failure is acute renal failure with very severe depression of GFR measured by the admittedly inadequate techniques we have available for measuring it.*

Dunnill *It does not explain the nephrogram, does it?*

Kerr *No I do not think it explains the nephrogram. Let me quickly pass this.*

Jackson *Dr Sherwood, have you anything to say?*

Dr Sherwood (London) *Well no, I just put forward this idea that nephrons are no longer just a nephron equals a nephron. The Homer Smith idea was that they are, in terms of distribution, very different and the outer cortical nephrons have a very different function from the inner cortical ones.*

Dr Shaldon (London) *Having come up from the same background as David Kerr I would like to ask a question. I think his suggestion that consumption coagulopathy associated with a miscellaneous group of non-obstructive renal failure patients could be associated with another* *organ, namely the liver. The work that I have been doing with some colleagues in Franfurt recently has tended to confirm that many patients in this miscellaneous group of acute renal failure which tends to progress to the stage of oliguria have, in fact, got consumption coagulopathy. Now the question is, which came first? The renal vasculature and the hepatic vasculature of the dog are not the same as that of the human and, therefore, with all due respects to Dr Sherwood, his excellent experiments do not prove that changes produced in the dog will result in the clinical syndrome that we are all faced with in humans.*

Kerr

Commenting on your suggestions about consumption coagulopathy. Obviously, it is a popular idea with us that it plays a part in the development of acute renal failure but, of course, it is very difficult to prove because consumption coagulopathy is such a common condition in many people who do not develop acute renal failure. Merely demonstrating FDPs in the urine or the blood or increased turnover of fibrinogen means that coagulopathy is going on somewhere. It would be very nice if we could prove that this was in the kidney, by counting the amount of iodine deposited there, but quantitavely I gather that it is pretty impossible to demonstrate it this way.

Dr Robson (Edinburgh)

I would just very briefly like to say how much I have enjoyed all the contributions this morning and there are just two points I would like to make. I certainly would not want to ask Dr Brun to decide the new term for acute tubular necrosis but, in so far as the tubules are concerned if you look at them under the electron microscope our experience is that you invariably see fracture of the basement membrane. Now this is obviously not necrosis in the classical pathological sense, but tubulo-rrhexis was a name that Oliver introduced from his teased out nephrons many years ago, and showed that tubules have got a fractured basement membrane. One imagines the kidneys to be a complicated layer of chemical and electronphysiological potential differences. One fracture in an intact nephron would disturb this, and I would have thought that this has or could have quite an important functional effect. One point I would like to make is that the urinary FDPs rise very quickly in the diuretic phase when the blood FDPs are quite low. Therefore I think that these products are coming from the kidney and not simply being filtered through the kidney from elsewhere. The other point is that the molecular weight of the urinary FDPs become progressively smaller and this does suggest there is a fibrinolytic mechanism in the diuretic phase which is associated with the return of renal function.

Dr Brun (Denmark)

Were your cases acute renal failure following shock or trauma ischaemia on the experimental animals? I can only say that on light microscopy you do not see tubular necrosis and in the ten patients which Steer Olsen studied he found no incidence of it and at least I suppose we can agree that what you should look for in the light microscope is not tubular necrosis. This is actually my main point. I do not have any explanation to offer why the kidneys do not function.

Dr Mallick (Manchester)

There is just one point that puzzles me about the coagulopathy story. In 1966–1967 Coles and I, in Cardiff, used the data processing system to look sequentially at a large number of patients presented to the unit there. We have data on 95 patients presented consecutively of whom 80 had apparently normal platelet counts on admission. Now, while I accept that coagulopathy is not always associated with massive thrombocytopenia, where we can clearly see DIC in renal failure there usually is an association and I am rather puzzled that if coagulopathy is the primary event in a large number of cases of acute renal failure we should in fact not find some evidence at least of thrombocytopenia. In fact the only correlation we could find was that the higher the urea the higher the platelet count. I wonder if anyone has any way of explaining how this might be?

Kerr

Perhaps I could kick off by saying that I think everyone would agree that overt severe disseminated intra-vascular coagulation is rather uncommon and I have shown you the ones that stick out; the odd patient with hypofibrinogenaemia of pregnancy and the child with haemolytic uraemic syndrome. But these of course are patients in whom the haematological changes are gross. It is possible that DIC is concentrated on the kidney where it produces quite small haematological changes. If one postulates that you have got a reduced renal blood flow through the kidneys as your primary event then secondly you have coagulation in the glomer-

uli, this may not be a big enough event quantitatively to reflect any changes in platelets or other coagulation factors.

Mallick *Yes, I accept of course what you say. It was just a matter of the primacy of the coagulopathy. I am sure we would all agree with Dr Robson's work and others that there is evidence of it but I was a little surprised that we could not find more consistent evidence.*

Dr Hall (Birmingham) *We have been measuring FDPs and also lysosyme in cases of acute tubular necrosis and also in patients who have been receiving cadaver kidney transplants and we found, particularly in those patients who have long oliguric phases, that the urinary FDP will return almost to zero levels several days before the kidney opens up and secretes its urine whereas the lysosyme levels, which are a reflection of a tubular defect, remain elevated until the diuresis is well established. I mentioned this just to suggest that perhaps we are dealing with several events here. Perhaps Dr Robson is correct that the fibrin platelets are likely to be in glomeruli but, in addition, there is a tubular defect which may account for prolonged oliguria and I would very much like to hear your comments on this.*

Kerr *Obviously I am in agreement with you. I think there are multiple factors involved. I think the attraction of this glomerular coagulation theory is that it also explains why you get tubular necrosis. If you have blockage of the glomerular circulation you will have damage to the convoluted tubules and I suspect that we will not come up with a single hypothesis. We will find that some patients get their diuresis as their tubules heal and some as their glomeruli open up.*

Dr Peters (Hammersmith) *I would like to comment very briefly on the idea that fibrin deposition in the kidney could be important in the cause of this and, I cannot help feeling that really a simple direct approach to the problem is what is required in the first instance. I think that what people are going to ask themselves is whether the fibrin that they can see in the kidneys of these patients seems to them to be sufficient to account for the development of acute renal failure and, if so, whether in the light of animal experiments when one* *induces a state of really quite massive intravascular coagulation with gross thrombocytopenia (quite unlike anything usually seen in patients) it is a common experience that it is difficult to find much in the way of alteration to renal function. I think that the measurement of fibrinogen turnover is quite helpful but may be misleading for the reasons we have gone into. The measurement of urine FDPs is also misleading because it is quite possible that, in spite of the work that Dr Hall just quoted in Birmingham, that the appearance of FDPs in the urine can simply reflect tubular failure, which, for all we know, the function of the renal tubule in respect of FDPs may be to catabolise them as has been shown to occur in other tubular proteins such as light chains, and I think that interpretation too has also been over-emphasised.*

Dr Joekes (London)

May I just make a comment. It seems to me a great pity if we lose sight of the very elegant and important observations that have been made on the changes in intra-renal blood flow. I think none of us working in special units will have failed to have seen the dramatic response 36 or even up to 48 hours after the onset of oliguric renal failure; having a dramatic diuresis and rapid return of concentrating ability by the tubules much more rapidly than you would expect, and all the experimental work which has now shown, for example with phenoxybenzamine, the ability of reversing this pattern of cortical reduction of flow. I think it is a great pity if we take what are possibly epiphenomena and lose sight of this work, and that we should be concentrating on trying to recognise the early stages which you can only do through urine characteristics so that we can learn how to reverse it and prevent the whole course of an acute tubular dysfunction.

Chapter 5

ACUTE RENAL FAILURE AND PREGNANCY

W.F. O'Dwyer

There is little new one can say on the subject of acute renal failure in pregnancy. Indeed with the exception of the description in 1968 by Dr Robson and his colleagues in Edinburgh of a new syndrome involving post partum cardio-renal failure in hitherto healthy women[1], little of note has been added to the literature on this condition in recent years. The present communication is no exception. It should be regarded simply as a commentary on our experience in this field since 1958 and with particular reference to the cases admitted to the hospital in the last five years. In the particular context of the Irish scene we are especially interested in the identification of 'At Risk' patients in relation to the likelihood of the development of acute renal failure consequent on pregnancy. Of 985 acutely ill patients referred to us for haemodialysis since1958, 97 (or 10 per cent) were obstetrical patients (Table 5.1).

Table 5.1 Acute renal failure admissions (1958–1972).

All Causes	985
Obstetrical	97 (10 per cent)

It is worthy of note however that in the first decade (1958–1967) the annual admission rate of acute renal failure patients in pregnancy was 8.5 whereas in the last five years (since 1968) this annual rate of admission has fallen dramatically to 3.5 per annum (Table 5.2). That the severity as well as the incidence of the condition has also diminished may be gleaned from the figures in relation to acute cortical necrosis. From 1958 to 1967 there were 13 admissions for this category whereas in the last five years we have seen only one case. While it is difficult to prove cause and

Table 5.2 Acute renal failure in pregnancy (Admissions per annum)

1958–1967	8.5
1968–1972	3.5

effect it is reasonable to assume that the improvement in this situation, both in relation to the incidence and the severity of acute renal failure in pregnancy is related to three important factors. In the first place the more adequate replacement of blood loss in an obstetrical crisis. Secondly, the improved standard of antenatal care, especially in relation to the improved attendance of women in the earlier months of pregnancy. Finally, there is the remarkable escalation in the use of the contraceptive pill for 'High Risk' patients. Failure to restore and maintain an adequate blood volume and blood pressure was a very noticeable phenomenon in the earlier years. Throughout the years under review we were fortunate to have on our staff a visiting gynaecologist, Dr Arthur Barry, who takes a deep interest in the problem of acute renal failure in pregnancy and who carried out a devastating programme of propaganda about this problem throughout the country. He had a simple formula: 'Estimate how much blood you think your patient has lost and give her at least twice as much as you think you should.

In order the better to examine present trends in relation to acute renal failure in pregnancy it was felt that an examination in some detail of the 17 patients admitted in the last five years might be of some value (Table 5.3). As can be seen from our list of associated factors, 11 of the 17 patients can be classified under the general and rather vague heading of 'toxaemia of pregnancy'. It should be emphasised that in all these cases the outstanding common factor was a severe rise of blood pressure shortly before delivery. Perhaps the most important additional observation to make on these factors is the occurrence of severe acute renal failure with toxaemia in the absence of any significant evidence of blood loss. One feels that the possibility of acute renal failure occurring as a complication of severe pre-eclamptic toxaemia, when no serious bleeding appears to have taken place is not sufficiently realised and therefore may lead often to a sense of false security and perhaps an ommission to observe urinary output

Table 5.3 Patient with acute renal failure in pregnancy (1968–1972)

Diagnosis	Number
Toxaemia	11
Hepatitis	2
Acute glomerulonephritis	1
Surgical trauma	2
Calculus anuria	1
	17

carefully in such circumstances. It is of course true that the combination of severe toxaemic hypertension and subsequent severe blood loss are by far the commonest precursors of acute renal failure and indeed in all our 14 cases of acute cortical necrosis seen over the years this combination was universal and obviously constitutes a very serious threat to the future of renal function particularly in elderly multiparous women.

It might be convenient here to make a comment on jaundice as a precipitating factor in acute renal failure. In our experience there would appear to be two different situations in which this might happen. There is a type of jaundice which appears to be a direct complication or part of the syndrome of severe acute toxaemia and it constitutes an added factor in producing acute renal failure. On the other hand, as we have seen in two cases in recent months, jaundice may appear in what is obviously an infective hepatitis situation and without toxaemia but in which acute renal failure may also occur.

The occurrence of classical acute glomerulonephritis in a 23 year old woman in the 38th week of her second pregnancy is of some interest. She was delivered of a live baby by a lower segment caesarean section but the period of oliguria was sufficiently severe to require three haemodialyses before the recovery phase from the acute glomerulonephritis commenced. It may be that the intervention of major anaesthesia and major surgery did contribute to the length of oliguria in this case. Her recovery was complete.

One of the cases of surgical trauma mentioned here was the classical one of damage to both ureters in the course of an emergency hysterectomy following rupture of the uterus. One ureter was tied and the other torn. Diagnosis was indicated by the immediate and total anuria following operation.

The second case of trauma was the result of an almost incredible piece of surgical stupidity in which a roaring pyonephrosis was explored with a finger in the belief that it was some kind of abscess. The exploring finger succeeded in splitting the kidney and giving rise to haemorrhage and bacteraemic shock. The patient, following transfer, survived miraculously in spite of the gram-negative septicaemia and the necessity for the emergency removal of the traumatised kidney.

The patient who presented with calculus anuria suffered a severe acute abdominal pain, anuria and miscarriage in the fourth month of her pregnancy. It is disturbing to relate that she was a 44 year old woman and that this was her eighth pregnancy. She had never had an investigation of her renal tract in spite of the occurrence of severe urinary tract infection and acute pyelonephritis in many of her preceeding pregnancies. The stone was removed by uretero-lithotomy. She had in fact extensive bilateral stone disease.

It is important to note the high average age and the high parity in this group of 17 patients and one should emphasise that this is a mirror of the picture in the wider experience of 15 years (Table 5.4).

Table 5.4

Average age	34.6
Average parity	4.8

Table 5.5

Maternal survival	14
Maternal death	3
	17
Foetal survival	9
Foetal death	8
	17

Fourteen patients of our 17 survived and three died. The foetal death rate in acute renal failure with us has been extremely high, as can be seen in Table 5.5, where almost 50 per cent of the babies died.

A brief glance at some of the important circumstances surrounding the fatal cases will emphasise how seriously ill these patients were (Table 5.6). In two cases we have the occurrence of very severe hypertension prior to the onset of profuse antepartum haemorrhage. It is of interest to note that the post mortem carried out on one of these patients (who died from what we think was a pulmonary embolus) revealed that she had in fact sustained a total bilateral cortical necrosis. Another patient (Mrs B) tells an old story which is still valid particularly among the itinerant class in Ireland. In the course of her 11th unattended pregnancy she suffered a severe antepartum haemorrhage and it was obvious that she had old-standing severe hypertensive heart disease which was in fact the true cause of her death. The death of Mrs C. in the first hour of her fifth haemodialysis is one about which we have some qualms of conscience although we are reasonably certain that it was not due to uncontrolled hyperkalaemia.

Nine patients of the eleven in the toxaemia group survived and one would like to make a few observations which may be significant on these surviving patients (Table 5.7). At a 3 to 6 months follow up, no evidence of significant primary renal disease was found in any one of them. Four of the nine however, remained hypertensive and five were now normal in all respects. It is of interest to note that the average age of the five normotensive patients was 31.8 years and their average parity 2, whereas in the hypertensive group the average age was almost a decade higher and the parity almost three times that of the normotensive group. Our criterion of hypertension in these cases was the persistence of a diastolic blood pressure of 100 mm Hg or more. We feel that it is reasonable to assume that these patients were old essential hypertensives rather than that they developed hypertension as a result of acute renal failure and it would seem to us that the presence of hypertension, even of a mild degree in an elderly multiparous woman, is the ideal setting for acute renal failure should toxaemia supervene.

It has already been pointed out that we have seen 14 cases of

Table 5.6 Maternal deaths

Mrs M. aged 27	4th pregnancy. B.P. 220/145. Antepartum haemorrhage. 1 haemodialysis. Pulmonary embolus Post-mortem – Cortical necrosis
Mrs B. aged 34	11th pregnancy. No antenatal care B.P. 190/130. Antepartum haemorrhage 2 haemodialyses. Atrial fibrillation cardiac failure. Cardiac arrest
Mrs C. aged 35	6th pregnancy. Pre-eclamptic toxaemia. Hepatocellular jaundice. Gram negative bacteraemic shock. 5 haemodialyses. Cardiac arrest

Table 5.7 'Toxaemic' Group (3–6 months following ARF)

Primary renal disease	0
Normotensive	5
Hypertensive	4
	9

	Age	Parity
Normotensive	31.8	2.0
Hypertensive	39.5	5.8

acute cortical necrosis in our series since 1958 and we felt that it might be of some interest to illustrate briefly the history of four of these patients who have had significant and useful periods of survivial as a result of regular dialysis treatment and transplantation (Table 5.8). In three of these four cases the necrosis was obviously not complete and it was possible to maintain the patients on conservative treatment for varying periods before they became dialysis dependent. The remaining patient had immediate and total cortical necrosis and required dialysis from the start. Fortunately however she obtained an excellent cadaver graft within a matter of months and is alive and well today with

Table 5.8 Acute cortical necrosis (Survival by RDT and Transplantation)

Mrs P.	
1967 (Jan)	Eclamptic toxaemia. Total anuria
	Regular dialysis treatment
1967 (Oct)	Renal transplant
1973	Well: Serum creatinine 1.5 mgm%
	Survival 6½ years
Mrs McM.	
1967	Pre-eclamptic toxaemia. Acute renal failure
	Congenital hydronephrosis. Solitary kidney
	Haemodialysis. Pyeloplasty
	Chronic renal insufficiency.
1969	Regular dialysis treatment
1971	Renal transplant
1973	Well: Serum creatinine 2.3 mgm%
	Survival 6 years
Mrs D.	
1958	Pre-eclamptic toxaemia. Acute renal failure
	Chronic renal insufficiency
1964	Regular dialysis treatment
1967	Renal transplant (Failed)
1973	Continuing RDT (Now deteriorating)
	Survival 15 years
Mrs. F.	
1965	Pre-eclamptic toxaemia. Antepartum haemorrhage. Acute renal failure. Chronic renal insuffieiency
1966	Regular dialysis treatment
1967	Renal transplant
1971	Died – Heart Failure
	Survival 6 years

virtually normal renal function.

Mrs McMs. saga is an interesting one: she suffered acute renal failure following severe pre-eclamptic toxaemia and it subsequently transpired that she had a congenital hydronephrosis in a solitary kidney which required pyeloplasty to relieve obstructive uropathy. In addition she suffered a partial cortical necrosis and the inevitable development of chronic renal insufficiency becoming dialysis dependent after two years. An added feature of rather dramatic interest in this case is that her husband became dialysis dependent at an earlier date suffering from chronic progressive glomerulonephritis. The husband and wife were on dialysis for a few weeks together, until Mrs McM obtained a transplant which has done reasonably well since. The husband is rehabilitated in his job.

It may be worth commenting on the graft survival in the three patients successfully transplanted on the basis of ABO matching only. Perhaps the absence of the inherent immunological processes of chronic glomerulonephritis may be a contributing factor in this relative success. The story of these four patients is not fundemental to a discussion on acute renal failure in pregnancy but one felt that they must be of some interest and in one case especially that of Mrs D who has survived for 15 years and is now sadly deteriorating, we have the story of enormous human valour and cheerful endurance.

To return to the broader problem of acute renal failure and to that aspect of it which we would consider the most important. We feel that the 'At Risk' patients in what is by far the most important group – the toxaemic group – should be identifiable. A patient over 30 years of age, with a parity greater than 4, in the known presence of hypertension and an obsterical history of toxaemia more than twice in her previous pregnancies is a 'High Risk' case. A few years ago we compared the incidence of obstetrical renal failure in over 800 of our emergency admissions with the incidence of obstetrical renal failure in over 1400 admissions. to the Hôpital Necker[2] in Paris. It is of interest to note that in the Jervis Street series obstetrical renal failure constituted over 10 per cent of the total admissions whereas in the Hôpital Necker it constituted only 3 per cent. The threefold higher incidence of post partum renal failure in Irish patients is closely related to parity and age. The average parity of the Irish patients was three times that of the French and in addition, the average age of the Irish women was 10 years higher than that of the French women.

Finally, some overall comments can be made on our experience with acute renal failure in pregnancy since 1958.

(i) This experience indicates firstly a very marked reduction in the incidence and severity of the condition in the current decade. (1968 to date).

(ii) A highly significant relationship with the social and cultural background in Ireland involving a relatively late age of marriage and high parity.

(iii) In association with high parity and existing large families a definite tendency for women to neglect regular attendance for antenatal care especially in the first and often the second trimester because of heavy domestic commitments.

(iv) A minimal, almost non-existant association with primary renal disease.

(v) With the exception of unusual problems, e.g. the hepato-renal syndrome and acute glomerulonephritis, an almost universal association with the severe acute hypertension of toxaemia. Essential hypertension, even of a mild degree, appears to predispose to the development of this condition.

The increasing urbanisation of Irish society leading to earlier marriage, lower parity and an increasingly enlightened attitude to contraception, especially in 'High Risk' patients will no doubt lead to a further substantial reduction in the incidence of severe acute renal failure in pregnancy – a condition which, in those severe enough to require dialysis, still carries a maternal mortality in the region of 20 per cent and very high proportion of foetal loss.

References

1. Robson, J.S., Martin, A.M., Ruckley, V.A., and MacDonald, M.K. (1968). Irreversible Post Partum Renal Failure. A New Syndrome. *Quart. J. Med.*, **37**, 423
2. O'Dwyer, W.F. (1971). Pregnancy and the Kidney. *J. Irish Med. Ass.*, **64**, 460

Chapter 6

ACUTE RENAL FAILURE AND GLOMERULO-NEPHRITIS

K. Peters, M. Boulton-Jones, J.G.P. Sissons, C. Brown, J.S. Cameron, and C.S. Ogg

Introduction

Acute renal failure is well recognised as an accompaniment of the glomerular disease, such as acute post-streptococcal glomerulonephritis, various of the idiopathic nephritides and the glomerular diseases accompanying systemic disorders such as systemic lupus erythematosus and polyarteritis nodosa. In this communication it is proposed to discuss two syndromes in which glomerular diseases are complicated by the acute development of renal failure. In the first, pathological changes in the glomerulus are sufficient explanation for the development of renal failure. In the second syndrome acute, and potentially reversible, renal failure which cannot be explained on the basis of morphological changes in the glomerulus, arises as a complication of heavy proteinuria.

'Crescentic' Glomerulonephritis

It has long been recognised that some patients with a clinical picture resembling post-streptococcal nephritis develop a fulminating illness, characterised by rapid deterioration in renal function resulting in death from renal failure. Ellis[1] gave a clear description of this syndrome: 'In more severe cases, particularly those dying with suppression after one or two weeks, acute fibrinoid necrosis of the arterioles and of the glomerular tufts is characteristic and early epithelial crescent formation may be seen. When death occurs after the rapidly progressive course, the outstanding feature is the formation of large epithelial crescents with associated haemorrhage into Bowman's capsule. Acute fibrinoid necrosis of the arterioles is common and a few cases show an intense inflammatory inflitrate of the interstitial tissue with 'explosive' lesions of the glomeruli and definite periglomerular inflammatory reation'.

The terminology of this type of glomerular disease is difficult. The term 'rapidly progressive' was used by Ellis to describe this evolution of acute post-streptococcal nephritis, but it is now recognised that the syndrome of rapidly progressive nephritis is not usually associated with streptococcal infection. The distinctive factor common to glomerular diseases of this type is widespread crescent formation. For this reason we prefer the term 'crescentic glomerulonephritis', by which is meant that the majority (arbitrarily defined as 70 per cent or more) of glomeruli show well-developed epithelial crescent formation. Detailed accounts of the histological features of this type of glomerulonephritis are to be found in the reports of Heptinstall[2], Bacani[3] and Sonsino *et al.*[4].

These patients present a major therapeutic problem, with irreversible glomerular damage leading to renal failure being the usual outcome. In recent years, the demonstration that glomerular fibrin deposition may be an important factor in the pathogenesis of this kind of glomerular damage (Vassalli and McCluskey[5], Naish *et al.*[6]) has led to the use of anticoagulants in these patients with some workers[7-9] claiming substantial therapeutic successes with these agents – usually used in combination with steroids and immunosuppressives.

In this paper the clinical features of 13 cases satisfying the histological criteria for crescentic glomerulonephritis are described and their responses to therapy evaluated. These patients have been seen since January 1970 in the Renal Units at Hammersmith Hospital and Guy's Hospital. A full account of these and other patients is to be published elsewhere[10].

The clinical syndromes associated with crescentic glomerulonephritis in this series are shown in Table 6.1. This glomerular histology was associated with a number of syndromes, but it more commonly occurred in an idiopathic form. Another indication of the heterogeneity of the pathogenetic mechanism responsible for glomerular injury in these patients was provided by the findings on immunofluorescent examination of the renal biopsies (Table 6.2); the appearances included linear deposition of antibody, suggesting fixation of anti-glomerular basement membrane antibody, granular deposits of IgG and C3 along the capillary walls and in some biopsies, only small quantities of IgM and C3. In no patient was there evidence to support a diagnosis of acute post-streptococcal nephritis. In only one patient (with polyarteritis nodosa and Wegener's granulomatosis) was the ASO titre elevated and no patient had hypocomplementaemia. In addition hyper-

Table 6.1 Syndromes associated with crescentic nephritis

1.	Idiopathic	5
2.	Goodpastures	2
3.	SLE	2
4.	PAN/Wegeners	1
5.	Relapsing polychondritis	1
6.	Henoch-Schonlein purpura	1
7.	Mesangiocapillary glomerulonephritis	1

tension was not a feature – the blood pressure being less than 150/95 in 11 of the 13 patients.

On clinical grounds, these patients could be separated into two groups. The first (Group 1, patients 1–7, Table 6.3), had no effective renal function at the time of presentation and therefore required immediated supportive dialysis; the second (Group 2, patients 8–13, Table 6.4) presented with renal failure but did not require dialysis at the time of presentation. In Group 1, three patients had an idiopathic crescentic glomerulonephritis unassociated with a systemic disorder or with any other histological form of glomerulonephritis. Of the temaining patients, one had polyarteritis nodosa and Wegener's granulomatosis, one had Henoch-Schonlein syndrome. In Group 2 there were two patients with systemic lupus erythematosus, one with crescentic nephritis complicating mesangiocapillary glomerulonephritis, one with relapsing polychondritis, arthralgia and progressive renal failure and two patients with idiopathic crescentic nephritis.

All 13 patients were treated with steroids, azathioprine and/or cyclophosphamide and 12 patients also received anticoagulant drugs. Arvin (ancrod) was chosen as an anticoagulant because this agent had been shown to interfere with the progression of experimental glomerulonephritis after the induction of disease[6]. This agent was used in 4 patients. Others received heparin and dipyridamole followed by warfarin (Table 6.5).

No patient in Group 1, i.e. those requiring immediate supportive dialysis, recovered significant renal function. Of the two patients in Group 2 with idiopathic crescentic glomerulonephritis, one deteriorated quickly and the other improved substantially. There was a high incidence of haemorrhage complications, with significant bleeding occuring in 5 of the 12 patients treated with anticoagulants. Bleeding from the site of renal biopsy occurred in three patients in spite of the institution of anticoagulant therapy being delayed for four to seven days after the procedure and gastrointestinal haemorrhage was the major factor responsible for death in one patient.

Table 6.2 Biopsy findings

Patient No.	Time to biopsy in weeks	No. of glomeruli	% crescents	Immunofluorescent Studies					
				C3	IgG	IgA	IgM	Fibrin	Pattern
1	22	28	90				Not done		
2	4	63	80				Not done		
3	4	10	90				Not done		
4	6	17	90	+	-	-	+	+	Granular
5	6	26	95	-	+	+	+	+	Linear
6	8	16	100	+	+	+	-	+	Linear
7	12	10	80	+	+		Not done	+	Linear
8	6	20	90	+	-	-	-	-	Granular
9	3	23	80				Not done		
10	22	22	90				Not done		
11	29	30	75				Not done		
12	4	15	75	+	-	-	+	-	Granular
13	3	10	90				Not done		

Discussion

This small series illustrates some of the problems that arise in relation to both classification and management of this type of glomerulonephritis. Firstly, it is clear that these patients suffer from a heterogeneous group of diseases, having in common severe glomerular injury characterised by epithelial crescents. Secondly, it is unusual to find evidence suggesting a streptococcal aetiology, although rapidly progressive renal failure associated with crescentic glomerulonephritis has been well documented as a complication of post-streptococcal nephritis[11]. The more usual histological findings in patients with acute renal failure complicating acute post-streptococcal nephritis is an acute exudative glomerulonephritis in which crescent formation is less florid; there are good indications that the immediate prognosis in such patients is better than in idiopathic crescentic glomerulonephritis of the type described here. The work of Habib[12] has established that crescent

Table 6.3 Clinical features of group presenting with no renal function

Patient No.	Age	Sex	Clinical features	BP mm Hg	ASOT u/ml	C3 mg/100 ml	Albumin G/100 ml	Diagnosis
1	14	F	5 mth joint pain, purpura and oedema	150/95	N	115	2.5	Henoch-Schonlein purpura
2	58	M	1 mth malaise, oedema and substernal pain	170/90	N	105	3.0	Idiopathic
3	21	F	8 wk post partum developed malaise and fever	130/90	N	110	2.6	Idiopathic
4	47	M	6 wk muscle aches, fever, depression and polyneuropathy	140/85	400 T/S-ve	100	2.3	PAN/ Wegeners
5	40	F	6 wk anorexia, malaise and vomiting	130/80	50	100	2.6	Idiopathic
6	26	M	Haemoptyses 5 yr 8 wk sore throat, haematuria and malaise	140/80	50	115	2.6	Goodpasture's
7	27	M	12 wk malaise, haemoptyses, shortness of breath and oedema	120/80	100	95	3.3	Goodpasture's

Footnote: N = Normal: T/S-ve = throat swab negative

formation affecting less than 50 per cent of glomeruli is usually compatible with recovery of good renal function. In attaching significance to the finding of crescents on renal biopsy, the extent of crescent formation must be defined and it is therefore important to obtain a renal biopsy containing adequate numbers of glomeruli. Claims for therapeutic success can only be assessed against the background of this kind of histological information; such information is rarely available in reports of such claims *(vide infra)*.

Table 6.4 Clinical features of group presenting with residual renal function

Patient No.	Age	Sex	Clinical features	Creatinine clearance	BP mm Hg	ASOT u/ml	C3* mg/100 ml	Albumin G/100 ml	Diagnosis
8	19	M	1 mth haematuria and oedema	11.0	140/90	N	90	2.0	Idiopathic
9	21	F	2 yr nephrotic syndrome (biopsy MCGN) 2 wk pyrexia, joint pains, vomiting	15.0	130/80	N	135	2.8	SLE
10	50	M	Otitis media, nerve palsies, haematuria, cartilage destruction	10.0	150/90	N	98	3.5	Relapsing polychondritis
11	6	F	6 mth sore throat, aching limbs and oedema	22.0	150/90	N	160	2.3	Mesangiocapillary glomerulonephritis
12	41	M	2 wk oedema, malaise	21.0	190/110	N	115	2.5	SLE
13	31	M	3 wk malaise and fever	8.0	120/70	Not done	100	3.0	Idiopathic

Footnote: * Measured as $\beta 1C/\beta 1A$

Table 6.5 Treatment and outcome

Patient No.	Predni-solone	Cyclo-phos-phamide	Azathio-prine	Heparin	Arvin	Warfarin	Dipyri - damole	Outcome
1	8	8	-	8	-	-	8	RDT
2	8	8	-	4	-	-	-	died
3	8	8	-	8	-	-	-	RDT
4	2	2	-	-	½	-	-	died
5	4	1	-	-	½	-	-	RDT
6	5	4	-	-	-	-	-	RDT
7	5	3	-	-	2	-	-	RDT
8	20	20	-	3	-	17	20	Alive 40 wk
9	78	78	-	26	-	50	78	Alive 78 wk
10	104	-	82	48	-	34	60	Alive 104 wk
11	44	-	44	8	-	32	44	Alive 44 wk
12	56	56	-	30	-	26	56	Alive 56 wk
13	8	2	-	4	2	-	1	RDT

Footnote: Numbers = duration of therapy, in weeks

In our series of patients only one of five patients with idiopathic crescentic glomerulonephritis and neither of the two patients with Goodpasture's syndrome showed any improvement on treatment with anticoagulants, steroids and immunosuppressive drugs. No patient in the group who presented with renal failure requiring dialysis recovered renal function. In the light of these observations it is of interest to examine the claims made for anticoagulants. Kincaid-Smith *et al.*[7] reported six patients, all of whom recovered on anticoagulant therapy. It is however, unlikely that they were treating a group comparable to the one described here. Evaluation of their patients is difficult because the extent of crescentic formation is not specified, but of six patients in that series[7], two had microangiopathic haemolytic anaemia, one had acute post-streptococcal nephritis and another (a girl of 14 who developed renal failure two weeks after an upper respiratory tract infection and who had an elevated ASO titre) is also likely to have had this condition, and one patient did not have crescentic glomerulonephritis. Only one patient possibly fell into this category. In a later series (Kincaid-Smith *et al.*[8]) four patients with 'progressive active glomerulonephritis associated with fibrinoid necrosis' were presented. From the information available it is unlikely that any of this group would have satisfied our criteria for crescentic glomerulonephritis. The patients described by Arief and Pingerra[9] seem to be more comparable with ours, although the crescents were again not quantitated. Impressive improvements occurred in two of six patients on anticoagulants, steroids and immunosuppressives. One was a patient with 'rapidly progressive' nephritis with granular deposits of Ig, C3 and fibrin and a second occurred in a patient with Henoch-Schonlein syndrome. One of the 13 children (Case 11) by Herdman *et al.*[13] was probably an example of crescentic nephritis and this patient also improved on anticoagulants and immunosuppressives. On the other hand, three of the patients described by Sonsino *et al.*[4] recovered on steroids and azathioprine without anticoagulants.

Assuming treatment had been responsible for the improvement documented in these cases and that anticoagulants rather than the other agents used, were responsible for this improvement, then the hazards of this therapy must also be considered. In our patients haemorrhagic complications were frequent and were fatal in one patient. Arief and Pinggera[9] also reported that all six of their patients suffered from haemorrhage and this was the immediate cause of death in one. Our experience is still too limited to allow any broad conclusions to be drawn concerning the value of anticoagulants in glomerulonephritis. Studies in experimental animals strongly suggest that these agents, given at the appropriate time, can markedly modify the consequences of allergic glomerular injury. But our clinical evidence suggests that when patient present with renal failure requiring dialysis, and the renal biopsy shows extensive crescent formation, anticoagulants are not only unlikely to help but their use is dangerous. If anticoagulants are to have a place in the management of nephritis it is evident that (i) some modification in the therapy must be made to reduce the risks of haemorrhage, and (ii) the criteria for selection should exclude patients with severe and irreversible glomerular damage.

Acute Reversible Renal Failure in the Nephrotic Syndrome

In the second part of this presentation we would like to focus on a relatively neglected clinical cause of renal failure, namely acute renal failure complicating the course of the nephrotic syndrome. This complication has previously been reported from Hammersmith Hospital by Chamberlain, Pringle and Wrong[14], who described nine cases of acute oliguric renal failure, four of whom had minimal change pathology; and a further three patients with minimal change glomerulonephritis were later published by Connolly, Wrong and Jones[15]. Since October 1969 we have seen a further ten patients in whom we have made this diagnosis. Since little attention has been paid to this condition, we thought it would be of some interest to describe these patients, of whom a fuller account is to be published elsewhere (Sissons, J.G.P., 1973 Acute Reversible Renal Failure in the Nephrotic Syndrome, to be published.) The clinical and pathological findings in the ten patients are summarised in Table 6.6. Two patients in this series died: one was an elderly lady with a previous cerebral vascular accident, who died of broncho-pneumonia and the second was a 63 year old man with ulcerative colitis, who died of a ruptured aneurysm of the splenic artery. Of eight patients who survived, renal biopsies showed that five had 'minimal change' and three focal proliferative glomerulonephritis. The most significant clinical feature of this group of patients was that eight of the ten had steroid responsive proteinuria.

On clinical grounds the patients could be grouped into two categories. Firstly, there was a group who exhibited clinical signs suggesting hypovolaemia. This occurred in five patients (patients nos. 2, 4, 5, 8 and 10); in three, large doses of diuretics had been administered to control oedema and it is likely that saline depletion resulting from this therapy was a major cause of hypovolaemia. There was a second group of five patients in whom no clinical signs of hypovolaemia could be detected; these were specifically looked for in all patients and included observations on peripheral venous filling and measurement of arterial blood pressure in the supine and standing positions. As shown in Table 6.1 the extent and severity of renal failure varied, with blood urea concentrations from 90 to 300 mg per 100 ml, and serum creatinine concentrations from 1.6 to 11.5 mg per 100 ml. In some patients it is likely that the blood urea values were exaggerated by the catabolic effects of corticosteroids. Oliguria lasting from two to fifteen days was recorded in some patients, but in others this was never documented. In general the urine sodium concentration was low – the lowest values recorded in each patient being between 3 and 36 mequiv per litre.

Table 6.6

Case No.	Sex	Age	Clin. Pres. to H.H.	Glomerular histology	Diuretic therapy before episode of ARF
1	F	46	Nephrotic syndrome	Minimal change	Frusemide 1 g daily for 2 wk
2	F	52	Nephrotic syndrome	Minimal change	Frusemide 240 mg for 25 days
3	F	40	Nephrotic syndrome and oliguric renal failure in a known case of SLE	Focal proliferative (SLE)	Frusemide 40 mg daily for 3 days
4	F	31	Nephrotic syndrome	Focal proliferative (SLE)	Frusemide 80 mg daily for 3 wk
5	M	16	Nephrotic syndrome	Minimal change	Frusemide 160 mg daily. Spironolactone 100 mg daily
6	F	26	Nephrotic syndrome and oliguric renal failure	Minimal change	Frusemide 80 mg daily for 1 wk
7	M	31	Relapsing steroid responsive nephrotic syndrome	Focal proliferative	
8	M	63	Nephrotic syndrome and oliguric renal failure in patient with history of ulcerative colitis	Focal proliferative	Frusemide 600 mg daily. Spironolactone 100 mg daily for 1 wk. Mersalyl 1M X 1
9	M	55	Nephrotic syndrome and renal failure	Focal proliferative	
10	F	74	Nephrotic syndrome	Membranous	Frusemide in increasing doses to 1 g b.d.

Oliguria (400 ml/ 24 hrs)	Maximum Blood urea (mg/100 ml)	Maximum Serum creatinine (mg/100 ml)	Sodium concentration during period of ARF	Patient clinically hypovolaemic	Outcome
15 days	300	11.5	21	no	Well. Renal Function normal
5 days	240	11.4	21	yes	Well. Renal Function normal
2 days	160		19	no	Well. Renal Function normal
	300		22	yes	Not followed up
3 days	200			yes	Well. Renal Function normal
2 days	90	2.1	11	no	Well. Renal Function normal
	150	1.6	39	no	Well. Renal Function normal
4 days	360	10.8	16	yes	Died of ruptured aneurysm
	260	4.6	6	no	Well, not followed up
	270		28	yes	Died of bronchopneumonia

Reference has already been made to the primary glomerular pathology. Examination of the renal tubules for evidence of tubular plugging by proteinaceous casts did not suggest that this could have been responsible for the development of acute renal failure. In some patients there was a minor degree of intersitial infiltration and tubular dilatation, but this was not a regular finding. Histological lesions suggesting acute tubular necrosis were not observed on light microscopy.

In four patients bilateral renal venography excluded thrombosis of the major renal veins. Intravenous urography carried out at the height of renal failure in one patient showed a persistent though faint nephrogram.

The cause of renal failure in these patients remains uncertain. The development of acute renal failure in a patient with nephrotic syndrome raises a number of diagnostic possibilities: renal failure may be the direct result of progressive destruction of the glomerulus by the primary disease process, or occur as a result of renal vein thrombosis or be due to the administration of nephrotoxic drugs. In this context frusemide[16] has recently been incriminated as a cause of acute renal failure, but the patients described showed evidence of drug sensitivity, including rash and eosinophilia, which was not observed in any of our patients. As has been indicated, investigations for renal vein thrombosis were specifically undertaken in the first four patients at the presentation. Subsequently we have undertaken renal biopsy early and this led to the demonstration of minimal change histology and the administration of steroids. The prompt response to this therapy makes it unlikely that renal vein thrombosis could have been the cause of renal failure in this group. No explanation for the renal failure was apparent from the study of renal biopsy. Certainly tubular obstruction by casts did not seem to be likely, nor did the radiographic findings suggest intrarenal obstruction as the cause of renal failure.

Thus some functional explanation seems to be the most likely cause of renal failure in this group, an explanation supported by the low concentration of sodium in the urine of most patients. The cause of this functional abnormality of the kidney is presumably related in some way to hypoalbuminaemia and hypovolaemia. Although the clinical diagnosis of hypovolaemia is difficult, especially in the presence of oedema, there was no evidence of hypovolaemia in some patients. Unquestionably hypovolaemia was a major factor in the development of renal failure in others. It is conceivable that hypovolaemia and hypoalbuminaemia, not clinically detectable, could have caused renal failure by producing an alteration in intrarenal blood flow, such as is thought to occur during acute renal failure in other situations[17]. In this context it is of interest that studies of the development of acute renal failure in experimental animals have shown that saline loaded rats are resistant to the development of acute renal failure induced by nephrotoxins[18]. It has been suggested that high renin levels may play a direct pathogenetic role in the development of acute renal failure[18,19]. It is therefore possible that high renin levels, resulting from low plasma volumes due to hypoalbuminaemia, might potentiate the effects of stimuli which do not normally cause reanl dysfunction. In this respect, the clinical features of our patients resemble the syndrome sometimes observed in patients with decompensated cirrhosis, ascites and oedema, who develop renal failure and in whom renal cortical ischaemia has been demonstrated[20]. The possibility that this mechanism could have been responsible in our patients is speculative, since we did not measure plasma renin or renal blood flow.

The main purpose of this communication is to emphasise the clinical importance of this potentially reversible disorder. In our experience this syndrome has been a commoner cause of renal failure than rapidly progressive glomerulonephritis.

References

1. Ellis, A. (1942). Natural history of Bright's disease: clinical, histological and experimental observations, *Lancet,* **1,** 1
2. Heptinstall, R.H. (1966). Pathology of the kidney, p.275 (London: J.A. Churchill).
3. Bacani, R.A., Velasquez, F., Kanter, A., Pirani, C.L. and Pollack, V.E., (1968). Rapidly progressive (non-streptococcal) glomerulonephritis, *Ann. Int. Med.,* **69,** 463
4. Sonsino, E., Nabarra, B., Kazathkine, M., Hinglais, N. and Kreis, H. (1972), Extracapillary proliferative glomerulonephritis; so-called malignant glomerulonephritis, *Advances in Nephrology* –(J. Hamburger J. Crosnier and M. Maxwell, editors) Vol. 2, p.121, (Chicago: Year Book Publishers Inc.)
5. Vassalli, P. and McCluskey, R.T. (1964). The pathogenic role of the coagulation process in rabbit Masugi nephritis, *Amer. J. Path.,* **45,** 653
6. Naish, P., Penn, G.B., Evans, D.J. and Peters, D.K. (1972). The effect of defibrination on nephrotoxic serum nephritis in rabbits, *Clin. Sci.,* **42,** 643–646

7. Kincaid-Smith, P., Saker, B.M., Fairley, K.F. (1968). Anticoagulants in 'irreversible' acute renal failure, *Lancet,* **2,** 1360
8. Kincaid-Smith, P., Laver, M.C. and Fairley, K.F. (1970). Dipyridamole and anticoagulants in renal disease due to glomerular and vascular lesions, *Med. J. Aust.,* **1,** 145
9. Arieff, A.I. and Pinggera, W.F. (1972). Rapidly progressive glomerulonephritis treated with anticoagulants, *Arch. Intern. Med.,* **129,** 77
10. Brown, C.B., Boulton-Jones, M., Sisson, J.G.P., Peters, D.K., Sevitt, L.H., Cameron, J.S. and Ogg, C.S. (1973). To be published
11. McCluskey, R.T. and Baldwin, D.S. (1963). Natural history of acute glomerulonephritis. *Amer. J. Med.,* **35,** 213
12. Habib, R. (1970). Classification anatomique des nephropathies glomerulaires. *Padiatrische Fortbildungskurse,* **28,** 3
13. Hardman, R.C., Edson, J.R., Pickering, R.J., Fish, A.J., Marker, S. and Good, R.A. (1970). Anticoagulants in renal disease in children, *Amer. J. Dis. Child.,* **119,** 27
14. Chamberlain, M.J., Pringle, A. and Wrong, O.M. (1966). Oliguric renal failure in the nephrotic syndrome. *Quart. J. Med. NS,* **35,** 215
15. Connolly, M.E., Wrong, O.M. and Jones, N.F. (1968). Reversible renal failure in idiopathic nephrotic syndrome with minimal glomerular changes, *Lancet,* **1,** 665
16. Lyons, H., Pinn, V.W., Cortell, S., Cohen, J.J. and Harrington, J.T. (1973). Allergic interstitial nephritis: reversible renal failure in the nephrotic syndrome. *New Eng. J. Med.,* **288,** 124
17. Hollenberg, N.K., Epstein, M., Rosen, S.M., Bosch, R.I., Oken, D.E. and Merrill, J.P. (1968). Acute oliguric renal failure in man: evidence for preferential renal cortical ischaemia, *Medicine,* **47,** 445
18. Thiel, G., McDonald, F.D., and Oken, D.E. (1970). Micropuncture studies of the basis for protection of renin depleted rats from glycerol induced acute renal failure. *Nephron,* **7,** 67
19. Powell-Jackson, J.D., Lever, A.F., Macadam, R.F., Robertson, J.I.S., Brown, J.J., MacGregor, J., Titherington, D.M. and Waite, M.A. (1972) Protection against acute renal failure in rats by passive immunisation against angiotensin II, *Lancet,* **1,** 774
20. Epstein, M., Berk, D.P., Hollenberg, N.K., Adams, D.F., Chalmers, T.C. Abrams, H.L. and Merrill, J.P. (1970). *Amer. J. Med.,* **49,** 175

Chapter 7

RENAL FAILURE AFTER RENAL TRANSPLANTATION

D.B. Evans

In uncomplicated live donor renal transplantation, immediate function of the allograft usually follows. Using cadaveric donors, however, experience is quite different, and in our cases more than 80 per cent of kidneys develop oliguric renal failure. The majority of cadaveric kidneys available to us come from road traffic accidents or from patients who have suddenly died in their homes, on the street or in hospital (Table 7.1). A relatively small proportion is obtained from intensive care or neurosurgical units where elective cessation of artificial ventilation is practised.

It has been well demonstrated that the following factors have an important bearing on the immediate post transplant function of a renal allograft: (i) the immediate premortem state of the donor; (ii) the warm ischaemia time; (iii) the cold ischaemia time: (iv) the method of preservation; and (v) the techniques of removal and transplantation of the kidney.

(i) An ideal donor should be under 50 years of age, previously in good health, who remains normotensive until shortly before death and is free from transmissable infection or malignancy. To have died in hospital whilst under observation would be an advantage, so that blood group, tissue type and renal function could have been assessed prospectively. Such donors are not common in this country, so that one often uses kidneys from less ideal sources. The majority of ours are notified by the local Casualty Department and are usually victims of road traffic accidents or coronary thrombosis. Such kidneys may occasionally give better early function than those removed from patients who have died slowly in hospital. Periods of premortem hypotension (treated with vasoconstricting agents) and poor renal function are common in the latter group many of whom will remain anuric after transplantation.

(ii) Warm ischaemia time is defined as the time interval

Table 7.1 Donor deaths

Traumatic	85
Cerebrovascular/neurosurgical	52
Cardiac	41
Drug overdose	5
Others	3

between the death of the donor and the cooling of the allograft plus the time taken to perform the vascular anastomosis. This figure takes no account of premortem factors. Several workers have found that if this interval is in excess of 90 minutes, post-operative oliguria is common[1-3]. We all appreciate the importance of keeping the warm ischaemia time as short as possible but there are many logistic problems. In this field one is dependent upon the goodwill of one's colleagues, nursing and theatre staff, coroners, pathologists and relatives. If there is to be elective 'switch off' of a respirator, all preparations for the immediate removal of the kidneys after cessation of heart beat can be made in advance. All too often however prior warning is not possible and the whole procedure turns into an emergency. Cardiac massage and artificial ventilation at such a stage has been shown to protect the kidneys from ischaemic injury and should be maintained until the time of nephrectomy[1].

(iii) Cold ischaemia time is the time interval from when the kidney is cooled until its removal from ice to commence the anastomosis. The duration of this period is not as critical as the warm time and one has seen kidneys recover good function even after 12–14 hours of cold ischaemia time provided the warm ischaemia time is short. The combination of long warm and cold ischaemia times however is undesirable for the degree of morphological damage increases markedly with time. Hulme *et al.*[4] showed that merely by surface cooling, successful preservation of the kidneys with warm ischaemia times of 150 minutes and cold ischaemia times of 600 minutes could be achieved with a primary failure rate of only 10 per cent. However, the longer the period of anuria, the less satisfactory was the ultimate quality of graft function. In a collaborative study from Paris[18] preservation of kidneys with warm ischaemia times of less than ten minutes gave 55 per cent immediate function if total ischaemia time was two hours and 44 per cent with total ischaemia times of up to 16 hours. Prolonging warm ischaemia time to 60 minutes resulted in no significant difference in the degree of ATN with total ischaemia times of up to 12 hours.

(iv) The continuous cool perfusion of kidneys using elaborate machinery has been shown to preserve kidneys experimentally for periods of up to 72 hours[5] but results in human transplant situations are so far sparse. Johnson *et al.*[6] and Kohn and Ross[7], using preservation machines, correlated the degree of tissue damage histologically prior to cooling with the amount of lactic acid appearing in the perfusate. Others judge kidney performance by measuring AV pressure differences across the kidney[8] and by the tetrazolium bromide test[9]. Collins *et al.*[10] showed that simple cooling using a solution whose composition approximated intracellular electrolyte concentration would preserve canine kidneys for 24–30 hours. Acquatella *et al.*[11] using a Collins C_4 solution made hyperosmolar by the addition of sugar improved the histological apppearances of preserved kidneys and Sacks *et al.*[19] using intracellular solutions containing mannitol demonstrated successful preservation of canine kidneys for up to 72 hours with hypothermic storage.

(v) The techniques used in removal and transplantation of kidneys are vitally important. Inexperienced operators may be careless in the removal of kidneys and may damage vessels and ureters with the result that the actual transplant operation is made more difficult. Traction tears in the arterial intima may lead to stenosis and infarction of the kidney, negligence over arterial branches lead to local infarction or bleeding and damage to the ureter and its blood supply can lead to important urological problems such as stenosis, sloughing and extravasation of urine.

Of considerable importance in regard to allograft function is the donor's state of health prior to terminal illness. Such information is often not available if the prospective donor is admitted to hospital in a moribund state. Relatives or family doctors may be contacted and questioned, and sometimes previous hospital records are available. However, as speed is very important at this time kidneys are often removed without any such information being available.

If recovery from acute renal failure following transplantation usually occurs within two or three weeks, why is it important to try and avoid ischaemic damage? It would be economically advantageous not to have to dialyse these patients post-operatively and the risk of post-operative haemorrhage during heparinisation might be reduced. Furthermore in any series of renal transplants performed in centres where ischaemia times are short and recovery of function is quick, the overall results are always superior to those of centres labouring under the problems of acute tubular necrosis. One important reason for this is the masking of other underlying processes such as rejection, infarction, obstruction, etc. Another likely factor that influences the ultimate outcome is the loss of nephrons that might result from ischaemia. This is hard to assess at the time and can only be inferred when and if optimal function is attained.

Causes of Renal Failure after Transplantation

These are:- (i) Ischaemic injury;
(ii) Acute rejection;
(iii) Ureteric obstruction or urinary extravasation;
(iv) Infarction;
(v) Septicaemia;
(vi) Dehydration and hypovolaemia;
(vii) Haemorrhage

In the presence of acute tubular necrosis it is difficult to be certain which underlying process is affecting the kidney. During this dormant period, occult complications can develop which may destroy the kidney. It should, therefore, not be a time for complacent observation, but should be used for intensive investigation to try and determine the cause of continued lack of function. Acute rejection may be reversible and it is probable that the sooner antirejection treatment is started the better the chances of its reversal. Obstruction to the ureter or disruption of the uretero-vesical anastomosis likewise need prompt surgical correction. Infarction due to arterial compression or thrombosis may well prove irreversible and require removal of the graft and withdrawl of immunosuppressive drugs. Complete cessation of urine flow would suggest an obstructive lesion of the ureter or complete infarction of the kidney, but where the patient still has his own kidneys, it is usually not possible to make the diagnosis clinically.

Isotop renography, urography, arteriography and biopsy may be helpful in differentiating these causes. However many other

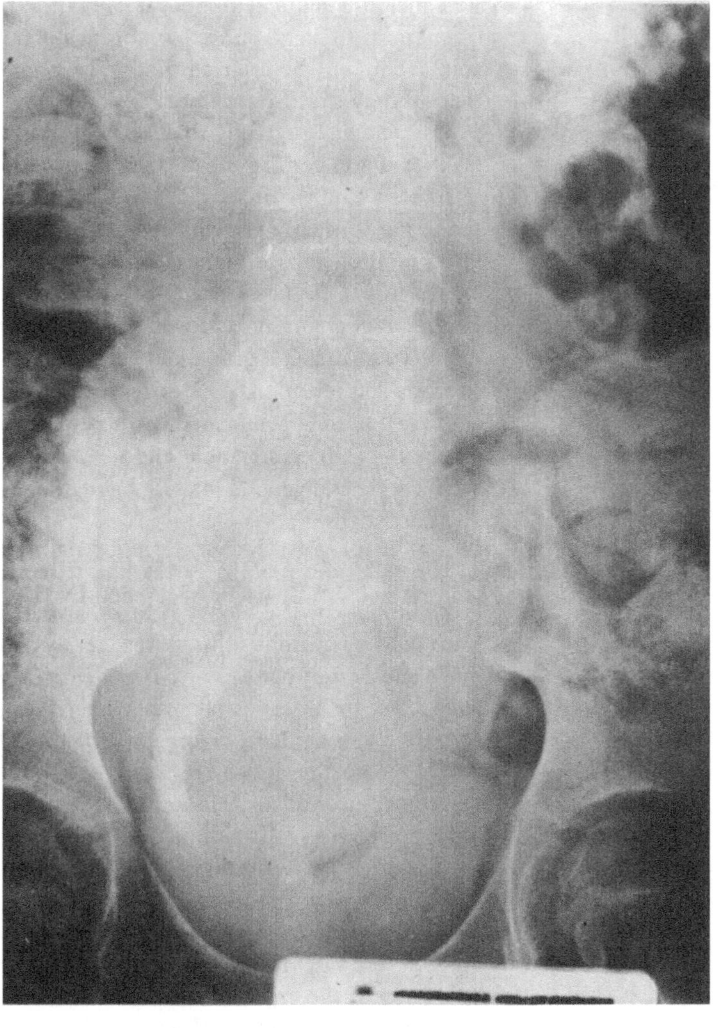

Figure 7.1 Urogram showing ureterovesical obstruction of allografted kidney.

indirect tests have been claimed to be useful, e.g. the uptake of isotopically labelled fibrinogen by the graft, measurement of urinary and blood fibrinogen degradation products, ultrasonic flow measurements, lymphocyte migration and complement estimations to name but a few. From the number of tests available, it can only be inferred that no test has yet been found that is absolutely specific for rejection.

Descending urography may be helpful in demonstrating urinary leakage and in confirming ureteric obstruction (Figure 7.1) but retrograde studies can be difficult with standard equipment for the ureter is usually implanted near the dome of the bladder. The interpretation of arteriograms needs a great deal of experience except in the diagnosis of an obvious main vessel obstruction. Isotope renograms have proved disappointing in that they frequently fail to differentiate between oliguria due to acute tubular necrosis and rejection. As Merrill[12] observed, the diagnosis of acute rejection depends mainly upon experience and clinical acumen – with enlargement and tenderness of the graft, fever, tachycardia and general malaise being the most common symptoms and signs.

The histological changes seen in renal transplantation have been reviewed fully by Porter[13] and by Herbertson[14]

An initial cortical biopsy is taken at the completion of the transplant operation – this serves merely as a baseline and too much should not be read into it[15]. In cases of anuria, a percutaneous needle biopsy is taken between five and seven days postoperatively or earlier if enlargement and tenderness of the kidney develops. Further biopsy is usually taken if antirejection treatment is unsuccessful. A functioning graft which shows diminishing function is usually assumed to be rejecting and does not require biopsy but if antirejection treatment is unsuccessful a later biopsy is worth doing.

Management is usually decided according to the biopsy findings. Severe vascular damage with fibrinoid necrosis or complete infarction of the organ would influence one to explore and probably remove the kidney. However, care must always be exercised when exrapolating the histological appearance of biopsies to the appearances of the whole organ.

Hyperacute rejection may occur in presensitised individuals and will only rarely occur if cross-matching of donor cells and recipient's serum is routinely done. However the titre of cytotoxic antibodies may fluctuate widely and the importance of using the serum with the highest cytotoxic titre has been stressed[16]. Failure to observe this rule lead to three cases of immediate rejection in our series. Septicaemias both with gram-positive and gram-negative organisms can cause allograft failure just as in normal medical practice but prompt treatment and dialysis support can lead to a successful outcome. Antilymphocyte globulin treatment can cause serum sickness nephritis and this was suspected in one of our patients who developed anuria, joint pains, skin rash and fever on the tenth day after live related-donor transplantation. A biopsy taken at the time however showed no evidence of this but *Ps. aeruginosa* was cultured from her blood and she recovered after a course of appropriate antibiotics.

Robson *et al.*[17] reported sudden haematuria and graft bed swelling due to rupture of arterial anastomoses in association with infection in six cases; in four of these the same micro-organisms were cultured from the blood stream of the recipient as had been present in the donor at the time of death. All the donors had been maintained on respirators for more than 72 hours terminally.

Ureteric obstruction or leakage have been associated with a high mortality due to septicaemia. However, with prompt surgical intervention, anatomical correction and drainage, the success rate has improved significantly. Ureteric problems may be related to poor blood supply either from trauma at the time of removal, from rejection or bacterial or viral infections.

Gross enlargement of grafts during the initial oliguric phase can sometimes be seen, and biopsy material shows interstitial oedema without significant cellular infiltrate or vascular changes. The exact mechanism of this condition remains a mystery but in our experience in three such cases exploration and nephrostomy drainage resulted in recovery of useful function. It is possible that some element of ureteric or venous obstruction might have been present which was corrected by laparotomy.

Conclusion

Every effort should be made to define the cause of acute renal failure following transplantation so that the correct measures are taken to try and reverse the situation. Meanwhile, full supportive measures must be taken to maintain the patient's health and caution needs to be taken in prescribing immunosuppressive agents and antibiotics.

If investigations indicate that the allograft is irretrievably functionless, prompt removal and withdrawl of immunosuppressive drugs is the only course.

References

1. Clegg, J.F., Kulatilake, A.E., Chisholm, G.D. and Shackman, R. (1968). *Proc. E.D.T.A.*, **V**, 264
2. Peart, W.S. (1968). *IVth Symp. on Advanced Medicine*, (O. Wrong, editor), (London: Pitman)
3. White, H.J.O., Evans, D.B. and Calne, R.Y. (1968). *Brit. Med. J.*, **4**, 739–740
4. Hulme, B., Snell, M.E., Kenyon, J.R., Owen, K. and Peart, W.S. (1972). *Brit. Med. J.*, **4**, 139–141
5. Belzer, F.O., Ashby, B.S. and Dunphy, J.E. (1967). *Lancet*, **2**, 536
6. Johnson, R.W.G., Anderson, M., Taylor, R.M.R. and Swinney, J. (1973). *Brit. Med. J.*, **1**, 391–395
7. Kohn, M. and Ross, H. (1971). *Transplantation*, **11**, 461
8. Slapak, M. (1971). *Transplantation Proc.*, **3**, 1547–1555
9. Maginn, R.R. and Hadjimichalis, E., (1968). *Organ Perfusion and Preservation*, p.505 (New York: Appleton-Century-Crofts)
10. Collins, G.M., Bravo-Shugarman, M. and Terasaki, P.I. (1969). *Lancet*, **2**, 1219–1222
11. Acquatella, H., Perez-Gongalez, M., Morales, J.M. and Whittembury, G (1972). *Transplantation*, **14**, 480–489
12. Merrill, J.P. (1971). *Transplantation Proc.*, **3**, 287
13. Porter, K.A. (1967). *J. Clin. Path.*, **20**, 518–534
14. Herbertson,B.M., (1969)*Proc. IVth Int. Congr. Nephrology*, 260–269
15. Millard, P.R., Herbertson, B.M. and Evans, D.B. (1970). *Lancet*, **1**, 113–116
16. Joysey, V.C., Evans, D.B., Millard P.R. and Herbertson, B.M. (1972). *Tissue Antigens*, **2**, 5–19
17. Robson, A.J., Evans, D.B. and Calne, R.Y. (1972). *Brit. J. Surg.*, **59**, 890–891
18. Lancet, (1972). **2**, 887
19. Sacks, S.A., Petritsch, P.H. and Kaufman, J.J. (1973). *Lancet*, **1**, 1024–1028

Discussion – Second Session

Dr McKenzie (Bristol) *I think we are all in agreement that obstetrics nephrology was established in Ireland. I would like to ask Professor O'Dwyer his views about dialysis during pregnancy. I just missed the early part of his lecture. I do not know if he mentioned what Goldsmith and some European and American workers have discussed – whether one can try and improve foetal survival by peritoneal dialysis and later haemodialysis or is it never worth doing? I just wondered if he had got any views about that?*

Professor O'Dwyer (Dublin) *We have only one experience of dialysing a woman during pregnancy and this one patient was a woman who had infective hepatitis in about the fifth month of her pregnancy and she had acute renal failure as a result of that and the results were good. She had about six haemodialyses. The foetus survived that period of about two or three weeks of total oliguria and jaundice and she recovered but, unfortunately, she did lose the baby some time afterwards. Whether that had anything to do with the incident or not I don't know. That is the only experience I have of that.*

Shaldon *In 1962 we had an eclamptic pregnant woman who was dialysed and I think in our ignorance in those days we dialysed her on an inadequately low sodium and exaggerated her hypertension and desequilibrium and by ultrafiltration precipitated a premature delivery of a live infant and ten days later on practically the same hour the mother and child both died. Now the point that seems to me of importance here is, would you say in your experience that, if you are dialysing these patients with hypertension and acute renal failure, are they more difficult to manage if they have had fits, and do they get more fits on dialysis in your experience.*

O'Dwyer *I think we always took too long to dialyse the patients. When we* *did wait too long and we dialysed them for too long at an individual session we had great problems there, but I could not be quite sure that they were specifically in the group that you mention. In latter times one dialyses earlier and dialyses for a short initial period and we do not seem to have that problem any more.*

Dr Blainey (Birmingham) *Our experiences are very much the same as yours. One thing I would like to ask you. Could you give us some sort of idea of the incidence of pre-eclamptic toxaemia in your material and do you feel that the reduction of renal problems in acute renal failure is associated with this? This is certainly our impression in Birmingham.*

O'Dwyer *I agree totally with you. As a matter of fact I think severe pre-eclamptic toxaemia or toxaemia with eclampsia is the major factor and if we can achieve a reduction in this particular condition I think it will probably remove by far the greatest cause of acute renal failure in pregnancy. The rest are just things that are unpredictable.*

Mallick *May I ask you two questions Professor O'Dwyer. Firstly, concerning patients who have established glomerular disease before they become pregnant. Dr Blainey has published and we and others have noticed they often go through pregnancy very well. Have you any contrary experience on this? Secondly, regarding patients who appear to be well before they go into pregnancy and then develop cortical necrosis; have you seen, as we have, severe proteinuria developing even though they are not requiring dialysis after the recovery or partial recovery of their cortical necrosis?*

O'Dwyer *At one time I would not have answered you as I am now doing. Yes, I would now agree with you and with Dr Blainey that if the renal disease is such that it does not give rise to hypertension there is an excellent chance of the patient completing a safe and successful pregnancy. Unfortunately however, people with underlying renal disease are probably more prone to develop hypertension during pregnancy. I think it all depends on the hypertension, that is my feeling about it. Your second question – Does significant proteinuria develop in patients surviving with partial cortical necrosis? Yes, though the amount is very variable. I think* *that some people with cortical necrosis have no proteinuria at all and some have a trace, some have a small amount and some have large.*

Dr Cattell (London) *Are you implying Dr Mallick that in your partial recovery from acute cortical necrosis you get a nephrotic type syndrome?*

Mallick *Well, we like to feel that we are giving them protein in the diet to prevent the classical nephrotic syndrome developing but I am talking now of proteinuria of between 5 and 10 g per day.*

Discussion after lecture by Dr D.K. Peters

Dr Moorhead (Royal Free) *Two points. One about the clinical nephrotic syndrome in acute renal failure which Dr Peters did not make (which I think he must have forgotten about) and that is acute renal failure in children, which is a well recognised problem related presumably to over treatment with diuretic therapy. I did want to also perhaps mention that, as he was describing it, there was a distinct parallel between his acute renal failure in nephrotic syndrome and the acute renal failure which occurs and is very common in severe liver disease.*

Dr Peters (PGMS) *I may not have made it very clearly, but I made it.*

Moorhead *Well, following on that. In severe liver disease it has been recently described that there is a very high plasma renin activity and I wondered whether there is local angiotensin activity in the kidney which might cause some diversion of blood flow away from the glomerular tuft. I wondered whether Dr Peters could comment on that.*

Peters *Well, we certainly have thought since we have accumulated the data on these patients about the possibility that renin could have mediated the acute tubular necrosis. As you rightly point out there is suggestive evidence that this may be a factor. Although I am not an expert in this area, I am not at all sure how hard the evidence is that renin is a major pathogenetic factor in the develop-*

ment of acute renal failure. We have made no measurement of renin levels or angiotensin levels in any of these patients and I am not therefore able to relate it to this disorder. I should be very surprised if the renin levels were not high in all these patients. The question is whether it is very much higher in those who develop acute renal failure than is normally the case. All these patients with a serum albumin are likely to have high renin levels. Of course patients who are hypovolaemic, children and some of these adults, can get renal failure for that reason.

Dr Jones (London)

In 1967, when Oliver Wrong was getting together the first cases, we had a similar one and we wrote up this patient with him and the subsequent history, which has not been published, may be of interest to Dr Peters. This lady presented with nephrotic syndrome, minimal change, in 1967 and had acute oliguric renal failure which needed dialysis for a month and then made a complete recovery and went into remission. Two years later in the same month she relapsed. This time she was admitted extremely promptly, she lived very near the hospital, so we were able to see her before she had even so much as a Bendrofluazide tablet leave alone frusemide or ethacrynic acid and we watched her very carefully and we watched her develop acute oliguric renal failure for the second time in the absence of any hypovolaemia short of the customary reduction of plasma albumin. She just got away without dialysis that time and again made a complete response to steroids. Her proteinuria remained highly selective. She has since relapsed four times, the proteinuria remains extremely selective, IgG albumin ratios of under 5 per cent. She responds very promptly to steroids and in 1972 she has developed an IgM para-protein with Bence-Jones proteinuria.

Dr Robson (Edinburgh)

I was very interested and glad to hear Dr Peters emphasise this syndrome of acute renal failure in the nephrotic syndrome which, I suspect, is increasing. We have seen several examples, and I think it parallels the incidence of the over-use of poweful diuretics and I think there is a tendency to use diuretics to the point of making people oedema free without considering what is happening to the blood chemistry. We have done a sequential trial using different techniques, infused plasma protein fractions or albumin with frusemide in such patients. One can show that if one does this one can give frusemide without causing uraemia, or alternatively, improve the uraemia without giving the frusemide as well as improving the oedema and I suspect that it may be too plausible, that this is simply a balance between blood volume and diuretics which reduce blood volume and, as the Glasgow people have shown, raise both plasma renin and angiotensin. One last point, if you do renal biopsies on patients with nephrotic syndrome with this degree of renal failure you can see evidence of tubulorrhexis.

Peters *Could I just reply to Dr Robson's point. We use precisely this regime of giving plasma infusions together with diuretics in patients where this syndrome seems to be incipient. I think one practical point which seems to be of interest, at least to the hospital administrators is that these patients do not as a rule need salt-poor albumin. Plasma with plenty of salt in it is very helpful. That of course applies to the patients who are clinically and obviously hypovolaemic and I do not think there is any doubt that some of these are related to diuretic therapy. I can show you some very beautiful examples of weight loss preceding the development of acute renal failure, but what confuses us much more, is the kind of patient that Norman Jones has described and several patients that we have since seen.*

Cattell *Could I use my privelege as Chairman to make a point at this stage in that we have had one patient, and this is obviously anecdotal, with exactly this situation and, being perhaps naive, we said that this was a hypovolaemic situation. So we measured his GFR using EDTA clearances, we plasma expanded him with massive human albumin infusions and got no change whatsoever in his GFR. However, when we subsequently started him on steroids his minimal change nephrotic syndrome remitted and his GFR went up. I think we may be talking about a mixed situation. There is something very funny about these nephrotic uraemics; it is not as simple as one believes.*

Professor de Wardener (London)

I think we have enough material, enough anecdotes, here to build up a good series. I wonder if all the people who have these cases have got the biopsies just when this happens because I have an anecdote too and it is exactly the same story. Minimal change, a woman with relapsing nephrotic syndrome which responds to prednisone, and every time she develops renal failure. I took a biopsy before and after treating her with prednisone and it is perfectly obvious that this is a tubular change. She has gross tubular changes before you give her prednisone and her GFR is very low and afterwards the tubular changes disappear. Now, alright this is one case, but we have enough people here if we were to get the biopsies together to show this.

Cattell

The point is well taken and personally I think that we are in a very fortunate position in Britain that all of us are pretty close together and perhaps if you take Professor de Wardener a little further can we ask those people at this meeting who have such cases to send the details of these to Dr Peters or Professor de Wardener or both.

Dr Platts (Sheffield)

I do not want to produce any more anecdotes but there are two types of this syndrome. If you accept that cases of tubular necrosis are not hypovolaemic, because they are overhydrated through not having any renal function; there is another very important group, which I classify as a medical emergency, and these are nephrotics which go uraemic without necessarily having received any diuretics, and they will develop tubular necrosis if their plasma volume is not brought up as a matter of urgency, with intravenous protein and if you are fixed as we are not being able to get blood volumes as an emergency, the only thing you have to do is the haematocrit. We have had patients with haematocrits of 60 and 70 per cent admitted with blood ureas of 200 and 300 and if we transfuse them with albumin they diurese in 24 hours, which is before steroids would have produced a diuresis. I think if you wait for steroids to work you will finish up with more patients with tubular necrosis.

Peters

Am I right in thinking then that this is a common syndrome or not?

Cattell *All those of you who have seen hypovolaemia and acute renal failure raise their hands up. 'It's common'.*

Shaldon *Why do you use steroids?*

Dr Robinson (Birmingham) *May I ask how one can correct this state without diuretic therapy? We have treated them by dialysis until they had a diuresis and then gave them steroids. I was going to ask Dr Peters whether he thinks that giving steroids in the oliguric stage does actually influence the course of this situation. The other point is the blockage of tubules that Professor Kerr was talking about earlier. The striking thing in what you were talking about earlier was the extremely low sodium excretions and very low urine volume and I was wondering whether this was a combination of a very low urine flow down the tubules and a massive amount of proteinuria. There might in fact be another cause of tubular blockage or something certainly interfering with tubular function as a result of this particular set of circumstances rather than just a hypovolaemic state.*

Peters *Take the first point. We give steroids to these patients when we believe on the basis of histological categories that they are likely to respond to them. This is our experience, and I think most people with minimal change nearly always respond and patients with minor focal proliferative nephritis nearly always respond. We would not normally give steroids to patients with minor focal proliferative nephritis but if we believe that the consequences of this disorder are life threatening, as they are in this group of patients, it seems to me to be a very reasonable thing to do. I think your guess about the cause of this syndrome is certainly as good as mine. I think I may have made it clear to you already. I am no expert in physiological problems related to the kidney and I appear to you in an unfamiliar role as a humble clinician.*

Cattell *Could I return to the earlier part of Dr Peters discussion, that is the acute renal failure developing in the patient with acute proliferative GN? Now I think the most important point he has made is related to the use of anticoagulants and steroids or some combination of these two. We certainly have had some of the same disastrous experiences as Dr Peters has had, and I think we have* *probably killed more people than we cured. What I am really asking is, is there anyone in here who would be prepared to stand up and say that this is the right and necessary treatment in these patients with acute proliferative GN or are we all still hedging our bets? I take it from you Keith, that you are a little ambivalent about this.*

Peters *My own view is that if patients present with 90–100 per cent crescents on a renal biopsy, and they are anuric, then there is no point at all in giving any of these nasty drugs. Now that is based upon a very small series of personal observations, but looking through the literature it is very hard, in fact, to find patients who fall into that category, defined histologically and defined functionally, who have done well. There are plenty of people who have described a necrotising glomerulitis, or something of that kind, who have got better, but not falling within these fairly rigid criteria. Colin Brown is responsible for the Guy's bit of it.*

Dr Brown (Guy's) *The group from Guy's with renal failure were not really acute renal failure, and still had some function. The difference between our group and the group studied by the Hammersmith was the type of anticoagulants used. Now by and large you used Arvin, and on one occasion I think you used heparin and Arvin. We have been using heparin and dipyridamole and I think it might be of value to think about the value of dipyridamole as opposed to the other ones that are mainly anti-fibrin drugs, whereas dipyridamole is mainly an anti-platelet adhesive drug and it is more the type of drug we want to use. This may be more likely the problem, or one of the problems, that is underlying this type of disease, although as you say, there may be multiple aetiologies. These two groups are distinctive not only by the fact that one was progressive renal failure and the other one was acute renal failure, but also the type of anticoagulant they received.*

Discussion after lecture by Dr David Evans

Professor Kerr *Does having tubular necrosis at Cambridge affect the long term function compared with patients who do not get it, and, if you were on dialysis and somebody offered you a kidney and the* *perfusion characteristics predicted it was going to have acute tubular necrosis, would you ask them to put it in or send it back to Bristol?*

Dr Evans (Cambridge) *As far as the first question is concerned, certainly over the period that we have been active we have not really been convinced that tubular necrosis for two weeks or so has seriously affected long term renal function. It may be that the over all standard of function may he not quite as good. I think the average GFR of those people with severe acute tubular necrosis ranges between 30 and 40 ml/minute whereas those who have not had tubular necrosis may have GFRs of 60–70 ml/minute.*

Cattell *The second part of the question you have not touched on at all David. This question of the perfusion characteristics of whatever machine you are perfusing with. Am I correct in saying that you do not use the Gambro or any other apparatus at Cambridge.*

Evans *Yes. There has been an awful lot of experimental work on preservation done in Cambridge, but we have never used any machine for human organ preservation. We have really no experience. We have one or two enthusiasts in the department, who are well connected, and who have been very anxious to start this going but so far we have merely used simple perfusion and storage in ice.*

Brown *Can I add one point about ATN. I have recently heard Karl Kelstein present this data from Minnesota on the long term survival of those patients who have had ATN. He found that in the first two years there was a difference, but over three to four years there was certainly no difference between those who had ATN initially, or even subsequently, and those that did not. The question I wanted to ask was in those patients who get rejections, do you think in addition they may also get ATN as well, and that there may be two things going on at the same time, rejection or acute renal failure, one of them immunological and the other one something else.*

Evans *I think this is probably true but I do not know how you would sort it out. I am sure that in some cases with rejection that there may be an element of tubular necrosis, if you would like to call* *it that, but I do not know how you differentiate between the two under those circumstances.*

Brown *The problem in management is always how long are you going to give therapy, e.g. hydrocortisone or methyl-prednisolone? How long do you go on giving it, or giving them radiotherapy, or actino mycin before they start passing urine. That's a worrrying thing in terms of the mortality related to giving these powerful drugs again and again and again for maybe ten days or two weeks.*

Evans *Yes, I get your point there. As far as we are concerned if a biopsy shows evidence of rejection the patient would have the benefit of a course of anti-rejection treatment. This may or may not result in an immediate, or within a few days, improvement in function. Now if it does not improve I suppose it means (i) that the rejection might be too severe and irreversible or (ii) that there may be ATN as well as rejection, in which case the ATN will persist despite the steroid therapy. Now, what we would do would be to allow the patient a period of anti-rejection treatment, which in say 10 or 12 days, he would be back to his original level of immunosuppresion. If no function had occurred at that time we would re-biopsy him. At that point if the biopsy shows fibrinoid necrosis or infarction then we would get the hell out of it and take the kidney out. This was not our original experience. I mean, we learnt just like everybody else by hard failure and we used to slam the patient with anti-rejection therapy four or five times in a month and they died but, nowadays, a failed anti-rejection treatment calls for a second biopsy and if that biopsy looks hopeless then the kidney is abandoned.*

Unknown Participant *There is one way of making a differential diagnosis of oliguria and that is a technetium scan. Although there are certainly a large number of causes of oliguria – I think the three main ones are infarction, rejection and continuing ATN, and if one gives a shot of technetium and does a γ scan with a computer output this can really differentiate quite nicely between these three different causes and this technique has the advantage that it is non-invasive. It seems to be very important these days in that it does not involve putting catheters in.*

Evans *Well certainly there was a meeting of radio-isotope doctors in Salzburg, I think they hold this every August, and there was a series of very interesting papers with this very point about the use of technetium and rapid γ scanning where they reckoned that they could even differentiate between cortical, medullary and pelvic concentration of technetium. We have a γ scanner but we have never been convinced that the resolution of the pictures was sufficient to give us very much information. I think Dr Joekes showed you some renograms this morning. We have a similar experience, but our big problem is that we can't differentiate on renography anyway between ATN and rejection. Fair enough if there is obstruction, you might get a different pattern, but there again, in ATN the renogram certainly looks very much like an obstruction or even rejection.*

Joekes *Surely function is more important than appearance under the microscope in this whole problem, and secondly I think that if you do renography regularly there is no difficulty in recognising the acute obstructive lesion, because this will show quite differently in the first few hours to 24 hours. I think that whether you have got a rejection due to immunological phenomena or primarily due to a vascular re-routing, is immaterial if you are in a position to follow the function of the kidney despite the presence of oliguria, and I think this is to me by far the most important in the handling of transplants, and has made an enormous difference in our experience.*

Dr Hall (Birmingham) *We have recently analysed the effects of the various warm ischaemic times on the incidence of primary failure and duration of oliguric phase in 100 of our transplanted patients, and we feel that the other factor in primary failure is kidney rot, and our evidence for this is that when the cold ischaemic time exceeds 550 minutes – that is nine hours – then the incidence of primary failure was more than 50 per cent. The initial warm and cold total ischaemic times were on average 26 minutes and 60 minutes. Now this was the same whether these kidneys were our own or whether they were imported, for the warm ischaemic times, but it is interesting and supports our conclusion, that the cold ischaemic time is very* *important in that 30 per cent of the imported kidneys failed to function at all, as compared with only 18 per cent of our own kidneys. So we feel that kidney rot is very very important.*

Chapter 8

THE PROGNOSIS OF ACUTE RENAL FAILURE

R.M. Lindsay

Introduction

Haemodialysis and peritoneal dialysis now have an established role in the treatment of patients with acute renal failure. As a consequence the prognosis from the renal lesion *per se* may be favourable. However, although the necessary dialysis and other supportive therapy may be readily available this complication of many serious medical, surgical and obstetric conditions continues to carry a high mortality, particularly in the surgical and post-traumatic groups. This reports presents the cumulative data on a large group of patients dialysed because of acute reversible intrinsic renal failure in Glasgow Royal Infirmary over the period from July 1959 to April 1973 in an attempt to analyse the factors which affect the prognosis of this condition. The report augments the previous communications from our unit[1,2].

Criteria for Inclusion in the Series

Acute renal failure is conventionally divided into three groups: pre-renal, post-renal and that due to renal parenchymal damage. The latter group includes acute reversible intrinsic renal failure, a term we prefer to acute tubular necrosis because of the lack of correlation between the degree of tubular necrosis often found on histological examination and the severity of the clinical course[3,4]. This group also includes conditions such as acute glomerulonephritis, systemic lupus erythematosus, bilateral renal infarction, etc. This surveyis restricted mainly to patients with acute reversible intrinsic renal failure. A diagnosis of acute reversible intrinsic renal failure was based on a history of a precipitating factor (e.g hypotension or bacteraemia), a period of oliguria in the majority (but not all), a low urine urea or osmolality, a rising blood urea, and a return to normal or only mildly impaired renal function in those who survived. The survey also includes seven patients with pre-eclampsia and four patients whose renal failure was subsequently found at autopsy to be due to extensive bilateral cortical necrosis. Their inclusion was felt to be justified in view of the similarity between their mode of presentation and that of acute reversible intrinsic renal failure and because of the view that a degree of cortical necrosis occurs in some patients whose main histological abnormality is tubular necrosis[5,6]. Excluded were patients subsequently found to have any pre-existing renal disease and those who had acute glomerular lesions. All patients were admitted to the Renal Unit of Glasgow Royal Infirmary with renal failure severe enough to require treatment by haemodialysis. The survey does not, therefore, include a further large number of patients with acute reversible intrinsic renal failure of lesser severity who were managed in other units or who were treated by peritoneal dialysis.

The Patients

Patients with acute reversible intrinsic renal failure can be subdivided on a clinical basis into obstetrical, medical and surgical categories. In Table 8.1 the clinical details of the patients are shown. There were 302 patients in total with a mean age of 42 years. There were 176 males and 126 females. The surgical group was the largest (169 patients), comprising 55.9 per cent of the total. This group had the highest mean age (51 years) and a male preponderance (ratio M:F = 3.3:1). There were 67 patients in the medical group (22.2 per cent of the total) with a mean age of 46 years and a male to female ratio of 2.2:1. The obstetric group consisted of 66 patients (21.9 per cent of the total) with a mean age of 30 years.

Table 8.1 Clinical details of 302 patients

Clinical Group	No. Patients	Male	Female	Mean Age (and range)
Obstetric	66 (21.9%)	–	66	30 (18–44)
Medical	67 (22.9%)	46	21	46 (17–76)
Surgical	169 (55.9%)	130	39	51 (9–82)
Total	302	176	126	42 (9–82)

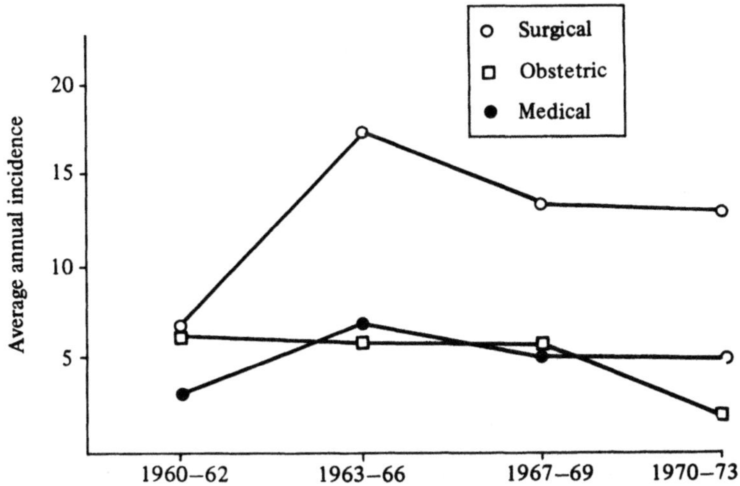

Figure 8.1 Mean annual incidence of acute reversible intrinsic renal failure for each clinical category from 1960–1973

Annual Incidence

In Figure 8.1 the mean annual incidence of acute reversible intrinsic renal failure for each clinical category is plotted for the periods 1960–1962, 1963–1966, 1967–1969 and 1970–1973. In the period 1963–1966 approximately 30 patients per annum were being treated; from 1967 to the present time this number has reduced to steady 20 patients or so. Throughout the period of study the surgical group is the largest.

Aetiology

The precipitating factors for the acute reversible intrinsic renal failure in the three clinical groups are shown in Tables 8.2., 8.3 and 8.4

Obstetric Group (Table 8.2)

Acute renal failure following spontaneous abortion haemorrhage provided the largest sub-group. Infection (in three cases due to *Clostridium welchii*) was a major aetiological factor in the six patients whose abortion was criminally induced. The miscellaneous group included precipitating factors such as hydatidiform mole, amniotic fluid embolism and hyperemesis gravidarum.

Table 8.2 Aetiology and survival (per cent) in 66 obstetrical patients

Aetiology	No. Patients	Survival (per cent)
Spontaneous abortion	21	100
Criminal abortion	6	67
Pre-eclampsia	4	75
Eclampsia	7	43
Pre-eclampsia + anti-partum haemorrhage	9	78
Anti-partum haemorrhage	7	71
Post-partum haemorrhage	5	100
Miscellaneous	7	71
Total	66	80

Table 8.3 Aetiology and survivial (per cent) in 67 medical patients

Aetiology	No. Patients	Survival (per cent)
Nephrotoxins	12	67
Pneumonia	12	60
Bacteraemia	5	80
Enteritis	7	60
Leptospirosis	3	67
Haematemesis	7	40
Myocardial infarction	3	0
Intravascular haemolysis	3	100
Miscellaneous	15	67
Total	67	61

Medical Group (Table 8.3)

Exposure to nephrotoxins accounted for 12 cases of acute renal failure. The toxins were sodium chlorate (3), paraquat (3), ethylene glycol (2), potassium perchlorate, mercuric oxide, lysol, and a multiple-compound plant fertilizer. Various forms of infection accounted for 27 patients (40 per cent of total). There were few cases of haematemesis in relation to its frequency as a cause of shock and it is noteworthy that the mean age of these patients was fairly high (59 years). Despite relative frequency of acute renal failure in the 'shocked coronary'[7] few of these patients apparently survive to a stage when dialysis becomes necessary. The miscellaneous group was caused by hypotension following drug overdosage, status epilepticus, subarachnoid haemorrhage, and steroid withdrawl.

Surgical Group (Table 8.4)

Multiple injuries accounted for acute renal failure in 41 patients, and constituted the largest sub-group. Various lesions of the gastro-intestinal tract provided the renal failure in 89 cases and in the greater majority of these a surgical procedure had been performed. The most common precipitating urological factor was haemorrhage following prostatectomy. Only four cases of extensive burns were admitted for dialysis; it is our experience that the majority of such patients die before dialysis becomes vital. The miscellaneous causes included repair of uterine prolapse, mitral valvulotomy, stripping of varicose veins, and clipping of an intracranial aneurysm.

Table 8.4 Aetiology and survival (per cent) in 169 surgical patients

Aetiology	No. Patients	Survival (Per cent)
Multiple injuries	41	50
Appendix, small bowel and pancreatic lesions	30	30
Gastric and duodenal lesions	22	30
Biliary tract lesions	22	31
Colonic lesions	15	47
Urological lesions	17	70
Vascular surgery	6	33
Burns	4	25
Miscellaneous	12	42
Total	169	44

Clinical Course

A total of 621 haemodialyses were performed on these patients giving a mean figure of 2.1 dialyses per patient. The number of dialyses performed in each clinical group is shown in Table 8.5 which indicateds that the multiple injuries sub-group required the most per patient. Fifteen patients required six or more dialyses, two patients (both multiple injuries) each having fifteen.

Two factors will determine the frequency of dialysis, namely the duration of oliguria and the rate of rise of blood urea. Ninety five per cent of the patients were oliguric and of these the mean duration of oliguria was 11 days (range 1 to 42 days). The mean rate of rise of blood urea was 40 mg per cent/day, 60 mg per cent/day, and 90 mg per cent/day for the obstetrical, medical and other surgical, and traumatic groups respectively.

In the earlier years of the survey dialyses would have been aimed at keeping the plasma urea below 400 mg per cent, but, latterly, our policy has been to prevent plasma urea levels from reaching 250 mg per cent. In the majority of cases dialysis was carried out using a rotating-drum artificial kidney of high efficiency[8]. It is likely that the use of this dialyser, with its membrane surface area of 3.2 m^2, accounts for a relatively low rate of dialyses per patient.

Table 8.5 Number of dialyses

Clinical Group	No. Patients	No. Haemo-dialyses	Mean dialyses per patient
Obstetric	66	96	1.5
Medical	67	125	1.9
Multiple injuries	41	143	3.5
Other surgical	128	257	2.0
Total	302	621	2.1

Survival

The survival figures for each group over the period of the survey are shown in Figure 8.2. The mean total survival rate in the early years was about 65 per cent, in the 1967–1969 period it was down to 50 per cent, while our current rate is 56 per cent. Throughout the period the surgical group have shown the lowest survival, those in the medical group occupying an intermediate position while the obstetrical type of acute renal failure carries the best prognosis (current survival rate of 100 per cent).

In the obstetric group (Table 8.2) the patients with spontaneous abortion had an excellent prognosis, all 21 surviving, while two of the six whose abortion was criminally induced died, in both cases due to *Clostridium welchii* infection. Of the remainder, those with eclampsia had the poorest prognosis, only three

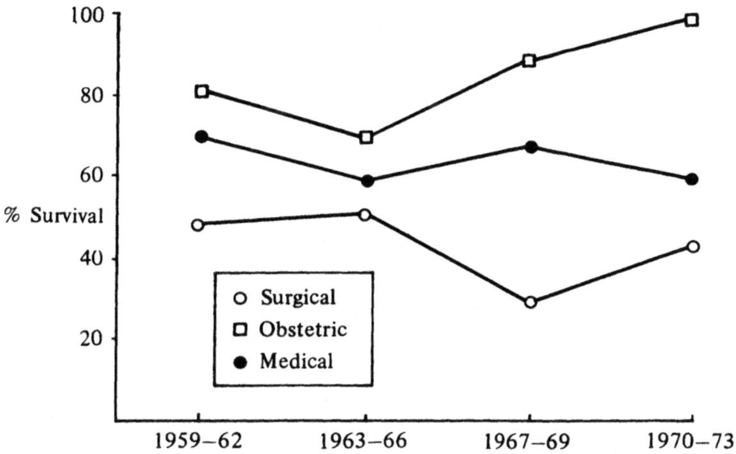

Figure 8.2 Mean annual survival per cent from acute reversible intrinsic renal failure for each clinical category over period of survey.

of seven surviving. In the medical group (Table 8.3) the patients who ingested nephrotoxins had a 67 per cent survival rate, the deaths being due to paraquat (3) and sodium chlorate (1) poisonings. The infection sub-groups had a mean survival of 66 per cent while all three of the myocardial infarction patients died as a direct result of the cardiac lesion. Within the surgical group of patients (Table 8.4) renal failure following lesions of the stomach. small intestine, pancreas, and biliary tree appeared to have the worst prognosis (only 30 per cent survival) while patients with urological conditions fared the best (70 per cent survival).

Primary Causes of Death

In 55 per cent of the patients who died death was considered as primarily due to the initiating illness rather than to the resulting renal failure or some complication of it. (Nearly 75 per cent of those patients were of the surgical category). In 31 per cent of cases death was due to common complications of acute renal failure such as pneumonia, septicaemia and gastro-intestinal bleeding. Miscellaneous causes relating to renal failure accounted for 10 per cent of deaths and included advanced uraemia (due to late referral), cerebral oedema with convulsions and cortical necrosis. In the remaining 4 per cent the cause of death was uncertain.

Sepsis was directly responsible for 40 per cent of the deaths; 75 per cent of these had severe infections prior to developing acute renal failure while 25 per cent acquired a fatal infection subsequently.

Complications of Acute Renal Failure

Complications, not necessarily fatal, were common and of the 302 patients only 70 did not have some major complicating factor or factors. These 70 patients represent 41 per cent of the survivors and thus the occurrence of any complication significantly affects the prognosis.

Infection was the commonest associated problem and was found in 55 per cent of the patients. The types of infection in order of frequency were pneumonia, abdominal sepsis, septicaemia, and wound sepsis. As expected the incidence of infection was highest in the surgical group (63 per cent). The next complication was gastrointestinal haemorrhage which was severe enough to cause a major problem in management in 36 patients (12 per cent) and in 20 of these it was directly responsible for death. Respiratory and/or cardiac failure occurred in 30 patients. Other, less-common, complications were hepatic failure, cerebral damage, wound dehiscence, fat embolism.

Comment

As indicated in the introduction, this report augments the previous communications from the renal unit of this hospital[1,2]. In the latter of these communications an analysis of the factors affecting the prognosis in 251 cases of acute renal failure is given. In this present report a further 51 patients, referred to us between July 1970 and April 1973, are added giving a total experience of 302 patients. Consideration of these 51 patients does not alter our previous impressions on the prognosis of acute renal failure and, thus, the reader is referred to the report of Kennedy *et al.*[2] for a full discussion. In summary, however, four factors were apparent which were indicative of a poor prognosis. These were:

Aetiology of Renal Failure

Figure 8.2 clearly shows the higher mortality associated with surgical causes of acute renal failure together with the good prognosis of the obstetrical cases and the intermediate position of the medical patients. Within the surgical group of patients renal failure following lesions of the stomach, small intestine, pancreas and biliary tree appeared to have the worst prognosis (Table 8.4).

Infection

Infection appears to play a dominant role in the outcome of patients with acute renal failure. Infection was found in 55 per cent of the patients and was directly responsible for 40 per cent of the deaths. Montgomerie *et al.*[9] in an extensive review of infection associated with acute renal failure confirms that it is a common cause of death.

Age

Considering the total number of patients in this series it was obvious that the age of the patients affected the likelihood of survival. The mortality rate rose after the age of 40, so that at 50 years the mortality is rather more than double that at the age of 30 years. This experience is in agreement with other reports[10-12]. It might be argued that the good prognosis of the obstetric group, who had the lowest mean age, influenced this finding. However, on considering the surgical group alone it was still apparent that those patients over 60 years of age had a much poorer survival rate (20 per cent) than those under 40 years (52 per cent). A recent report from the Belfast group[13] suggested that the prognosis of elderly patients with acute renal failure was not different from others. In that series, however, the majority of the patients did not appear to have established acute reversible intrinsic renal failure as many responded to correction of electrolyte and fluid balance disorders and dialysis was only required in 24.6 per cent of the total. We would agree that elderly patients with pre-renal renal failure do well with correct and prompt management.

Gastrointestinal Bleeding

Gastrointestinal haemorrhage occurred in 36 per cent of the patients and in 20 of these it was directly responsible for death. This complication was commonest in the surgical cases but also occurred in a proportion of the medical cases. In a few cases the haemorrhage was a direct consequence of the initial illness, e.g. peptic ulcer but in many it was regarded solely as a complication of renal failure. A quantitative and qualitative defect in platelets[14] may be a factor in this bleeding tendency.

An overall survival rate of 56 per cent at the present time is, in our opinion, still depressingly low. There have been dramatic advances in the treatment of chronic renal failure in recent years yet we have not improved the prognosis of acute reversible intrinsic renal failure in 13 years (Figure 8.2). The likely reason for this is a shift in the spectrum of severity of the syndrome of acute reversible intrinsic renal failure. On the one hand the greater awareness of the possibility of renal failure in the 'at risk' situation together with the prompt correction of adverse features such as hypovolaemia prevents many patients (who previously would have required treatment) from developing established renal failure. At the other end of the spectrum major surgery is being performed on 'poor risk' patients in the older age groups and who are, now, surviving long enough to require treatment for their subsequent acute renal failure. This opinion is shared by Stott *et al.*[15]. Considerable effort by clinicians experienced in the management of patients with acute renal failure is still required if we are to improve the prognosis of this condition.

Acknowledgements This survey reflects the work of a large number of clinicians and nurses who have worked, over the years, in the Renal Unit under Professor A.C. Kennedy's direction. This report is presented on their behalf with the permission of Professor Kennedy.

References

1. Kennedy, A.C., Luke, R.G., Linton, A.L., Eaton, J.C. and Gray, M.J.B. (1963). *Scot. Med. J.*, **8**, 97
2. Kennedy, A.C., Burton, J.A., Luke, R.G., Briggs, J.D., Lindsay, R.M., Allison, M.E.M., Edward, N. and Dargie, H.J., (1973). *Quart. J. Med.*, **42**, 165, 73.
3. Sevitt, S. (1959). *Lancet*, **2**, 135
4. Finckh, E.S., Jeremy, D. and Whyte, H.M. (1962). *Quart. J. Med.*, **31**, 429
5. Swann, R.C. and Merrill, J.P. (1953). *Medicine (Baltimore)*, **32**, 215
6. Lauler, D. and Schreiner, G.E. (1958). *Amer. J. Med.*, **24**, 519
7. Hutton, I., Pack, A.I., Lindsay, R.M. and Lawrie, T.D.V. (1970). *Lancet*, **2**, 123
8. Kennedy, A.C., Gray, M.J.B., Dinwoodie, A. and Linton, A.L. (1961). *Lancet*, 966
9. Mongomerie, J.Z., Kalnanson, G.M. and Guze, L.B. (1968). *Medicine (Baltimore)*, **47**, 1
10. Kiley, J.E., Jowers, S.R. and Beebe, R.T. (1960). *New Eng. J. Med.*, **262**, 481
11. Balslov, J.T. and Jorgensen, H.E. (1963). *Amer. J. Med.*, **34**, 753
12. Eales, L., Dowdle, E.B. and Saunders, S.J. (1964). *South Afr. Med. J.*, **38**, 251
13. Kumar, R., Hill, C.M and McGeown, M.G. (1973). *Lancet*, **1**, 90
14. Stewart, J.H. and Castaldi, P.A. (1967). *Quart. J. Med.*, **36**, 409
15. Stott, R.B., Cameron, J.S., Ogg, C.S. and Bewick, M.(1972). *Lancet* **2**, 75

Chapter 9

TREATMENT OF ACUTE RENAL FAILURE

C.T. Flynn

The first part of this paper deals briefly with selected aspects of the treatment of acute renal failure. These are drawn largely from our experience at Princess Mary's R.A.F. Hospital, Halton, and are intended to highlight both progress and problems. The second part is a presentation of the results of the questionnaire described in the Introduction.

In the treatment of acute renal failure it is useful to consider the renal lesion, the renal failure and the associated disease separately. This allows a more orderly approach to the assessment of priorities, remembering of course that they are all inter-related.

Treatment of Renal Lesion

It is obvious that the nephrologist has most to offer in the diagnosis and treatment of the renal lesion. A partial list of the main diagnoses which need to be of systemically examined in all cases is given in Table 9.1, as well as the main aids to diagnosis in order of importance. Space does not permit a detailed discussion but some are worthy of special mention.

Diuretics

The use of diuretics in pre-renal failure is controversial. It is not well known that diuresis following rehydration may be delayed by several hours. Diuretics may hasten diuresis but this is not proof that diuresis would not have occurred. Occasionally an increase in urine volume may occur without improvement in renal function. We are seeing more frequently oliguria ensuing late in the course of a serious complicated illness. In our experience diuretics never work in this situation, even though eventual recovery or renal function may occur.

Chronic Renal Failure

The diagnosis of chronic renal disease is crucial to prognosis. Mistakes can be made in either direction, but if in doubt it is better to assume that failure is acute and wait on events. Fear of

Table 9.1 Treatment of renal lesion

Aids	Diagnosis
History	Pre-renal
Examination	Post-renal
Laboratory	Intrinsic
Radiology	Nephrotoxic
	Nephritic
	Vascular
Biopsy	Chronic

having to place a patient on a chronic dialysis programme should not be allowed to inhibit treatment.

Renal Biopsy

This is often unnecessary but may occasionally be essential, as in rapidly progressive glomerulonephritis. If so, urgent measures are required to discover the size and position of kidneys,,cure the uraemic bleeding tendency by dialysis and make the patient alert and co-operative. If there is little doubt that the patient has acute intrinsic renal failure the urgency of treatment can be judged on strict clinical grounds, and biopsy avoided.

Radiology

A good quality high dose intravenous urogram is most useful in excluding obstruction. We have seen cases of acute intrinsic renal failure in which the immediate dense, persistent nephrogram described by Fry[1] does not occur. This investigation is time consuming and may be very difficult to perform. It is carried out on most of our patients but not until the patient has improved and has a stable blood pressure.

Treatment of Associated Disease

The treatment of the associated disease is strongly influenced by the co-existence of renal failure and some of the more important aspects are shown in Table 9.2.

Drugs such as water-soluble vitamins and antibiotics may be lost during dialysis. Toxic antibiotics which are excreted by the kidney, such as gentamycin, may have to be given in modified dosage and blood levels monitored to ensure adequacy and prevent toxicity. Nephrotoxic drugs, such as colistin, must be avoided and catabolic drugs, such as tetracycline, may increase the

Table 9.2 Treatment of associate disease

Drugs	Dialysis Toxic, excreted by kidney Nephrotoxic Catabolic Soporific
Surgery	Debridement Pre- / Post- operative dialysis Anaesthesia
Nutrition	Hypercatabolic patients Need high calorie intake Dialysis losses of amino acids and vitamins need replacement

uraemic problem. Soporific drugs can cause confusion with uraemia and in our experience intravenous diazepam (Valium) is short lived and safe.

The commonest cause of death in acute renal failure is septicaemia and a focus of necrotic tissue is a very adverse factor in prognosis. Debridement is therefore mandatory, although it must be admitted that this is a counsel of perfection and often poses a difficult therapeutic dilemma.

Surgical procedures of all kinds may be needed and dialysis will be required before operation and often afterwards. Anaesthesia must be given with very adequate ventilation (and a minimum of drugs).

Lastly, the importance of adequate nutrition in hypercatabolic patients needs to be stressed. Patients will burn up their own flesh unless given adequate calories, thus increasing morbidity, jeopardising survival and prolonging convalescence. Intravenous amino acids are necessary to replace dialysis losses. The provision of calories and amino acids requires a volume and this is not available in an oliguric patient unless it is obtained by volume removal at dialyis. The provision of calories is the most cogent reason for frequent dialysis and should take precedence over biochemical or other parameters.

Table 9.3 Indications for dialysis

Peritoneal	Haemodialysis
1. Acute on chronic renal failure	1. Hypercatabolism
2. Associated heart failure	2. Abdominal conditions contra-indicating peritoneal dialysis
3. Children	
4. Haemolytic anaemia	
5. Haemorrhage states	

Treatment of Renal Failure

This section is mainly concerned with dialysis. The choice is between peritoneal dialysis and haemodialysis. The former is simple, requiring only a catheter passed into the peritoneal cavity which is then irrigated continually or intermittently by a warm, sterile physiological solution made hypertonic with dextrose. It is very useful for the removal of excess fluid from the body but is much less efficient than haemodialysis in the removal of retained nitrogenous products. Haemodialysis requires access to the blood stream with either an arterio-venous shunt or a catheter placed in the inferior vena cava[2]. It requires special skills of a sort that must be practiced frequently and has evolved into a remarkably simple procedure because of the demands of chronic dialysis. There is little difference in the cost of either procedure. In practise the choice between them exists only when both are available otherwise the choice is really between treating with peritoneal dialysis or transferring the patient to a renal unit. Our own unit does offer a mobile service, when possible, in which a team will take an artificial kidney to treat a patient who cannot be moved. Because there is a natural reluctance to transfer patients and because renal units are overworked it may often be that peritoneal dialysis is chosen for convenience, or by necessity, rather than by consideration of specific criteria as listed in Table 9.3. They are reasonably self evident and will not be discussed further. One can actually combine both techniques by placing two catheters in the peritoneal cavity and redialysing the peritoneal fluid through an artificial kidney, as shown in Figure 9.1. It is simple, quite effective and avoids protein loss but is something of a medical curiosity.

Many patients can, of course, be treated by either method and in the absence of specific indications the choice can be made on

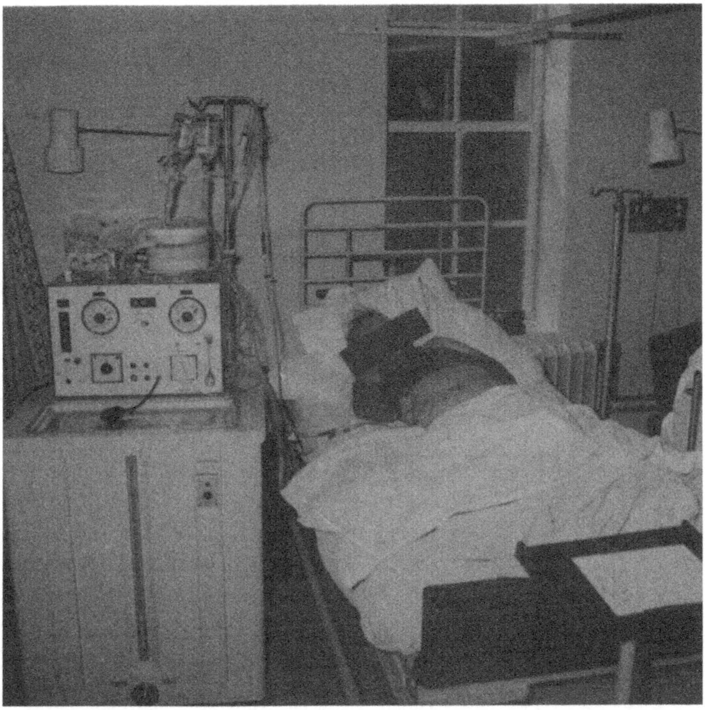

Figure 9.1 The patient has two silastic peritoneal catheters *in situ*. The peritoneal fluid is being recirculated through a coil haemodialyser. The dialysis fluid contains a high concentration of dextrose to prevent a loss of dextrose from the peritoneal fluid.

more general considerations. It is the severity, of the associated disease, particularly infection and traumatised tissue, which determines the degree of catabolism and hence the need for dialysis. The success of peritoneal dialysis, despite its relative inefficiency is, in my view, largely related to the provision of calories that it allows. However, in hypercatabolic situations, where the calories are most needed, it provides inadequate control of the uraemia. The duration of renal failure is a more important factor than the degree which, in the majority of cases, is for practical purposes complete while it lasts. These points are summarised in Table 9.4.

Table 9.4 Duration of renal failure

Severity of Associated Disease	Mild	Moderate	Severe
Mild	C	P	H
Moderate	P	P	H
Severe	H	H	H

Footnote: C = Conservative; P = Peritoneal dialysis; H = Haemodialysis

Case Report

Some points illustrating technological advance in haemodialysis are given in the following case report. The patient had a total colectomy and ileostomy for ulcerative colitis late in 1972. In February 1973 obstruction of the ileostomy occurred and this was corrected by operation. Cellulitis of the abdominal wall developed causing necrosis of skin and subcutaneous tissue down to muscle. Virtually the whole of the abdominal wall was involved except, fortunately, around the ileostomy. The patient then developed acute renal failure, and was hypercatabolic. Peritoneal dialysis was contra-indicated. Parenteral feeding (including blood and albumin) was essential and this was given through a wide-bore Teflon catheter inserted into the inferior vena cava via the right femoral vein. Daily haemodialysis was performed for six hours using a modern small volume dialyser. In addition an apparatus (Unipuncture system, Vital Assists Corporation) was used which allows dialysis through a single needle[3] (Figure 9.2). The Teflon catheter, dialyser and unipuncture system have all been developed for the dialysis of chronic renal failure patients and would otherwise not exist. To dialyse the patient it was only necessary to disconnect the unipuncture system. The whole procedure was painless and produced no haemodynamic disturbance or symptoms of any sort.

Debridement of the abdominal wall was achieved and a skin graft was applied which completely healed while the patient was in renal failure. Two weeks after dialysis was discontinued the patient was completely well and at home. While this case illustrates the efficiency and simplicity of haemodialysis it must be remembered that the severity of the associated disease is still

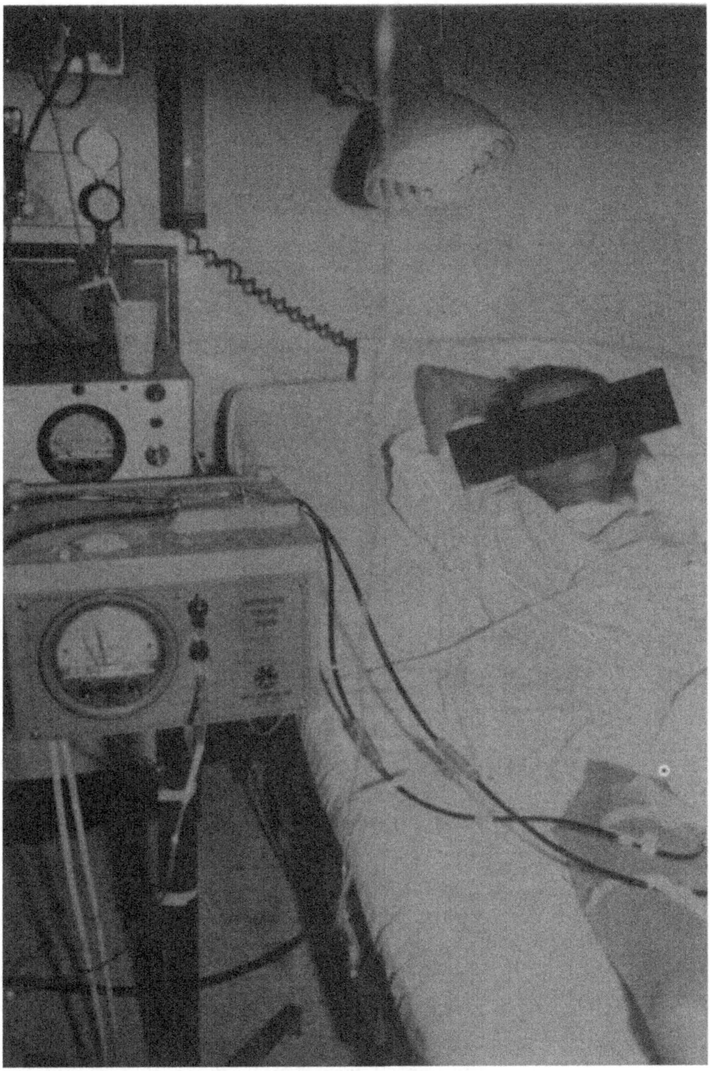

Figure 9.2 The patient has a single Teflon catheter lying in the inferior vena cava having been inserted through the right femoral vein. This is connected by tubing passing through a 'Unipuncture System' apparatus which avoids the need for venepuncture to allow return flow of blood. The haemodialyser is not shown.

Table 9.5

Patients		20
Survivors		17
Ages		17- 68 yrs
	Average	31 yrs
Duration of oliguria		6–30 days
	Average	22.6
Average blood urea before first dialysis		360 mg %
Total Dialysis		271
	Average per patient	13.5

the major determinant of mortality[4]. Unfortunately, the proportion of seriously ill patients seems to be increasing both in our experience and that of others[5]. It is difficult to decide on the value of frequent haemodialysis in the most seriously ill patients and pessimism has been expressed, particularly in the paper from Guy's Hospital. That it is of value seems to us to be most clearly demonstrable in accidental trauma, perhaps because this group usually contains the most profoundly hypercatabolic patients.

Table 9.5 shows our first 20 patients with accidental trauma (excluding burns) treated from the time we began to use frequent (daily) haemodialysis in 1965. It can be seen that they were severely uraemic at the time of the first dialysis, had prolonged oliguria, and received a lot of haemodialysis. Their injuries were severe, and included a considerable number of intra-abdominal injuries (Table 9.6) usually considered to carry a worse prognosis than limb or thoracic injuries. Seventeen of these patients survived. The next 19 patients had a worse mortality rate, mainly because we were treating ever increasingly injured patients, but the overall mortality of these 39 patients was 36 per cent, a figure which is below the national average for all forms of acute renal failure.

With the passing of time there has been an increasing demand from civilian intensive care units. In the early period 1965–1967 (Table 9.7) the mortality rate of patients admitted to the renal unit and those treated by mobile dialysis were almost identical.

Table 9.6 Intra-abdominal injuries among survivors (20 cases of trauma)

2	Lacerated livers
3	Lacerated kidneys (all lost)
2	Ruptured spleens
1	Transected small bowel
4	Perforations small bowel
1	Perforation of rectum

Table 9.7

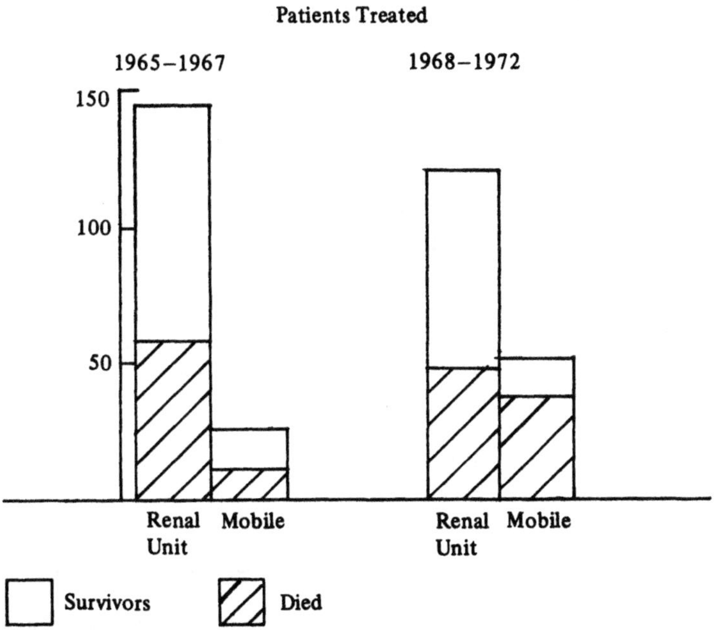

During the second period 1968–1972 there is a decline in total admissions to the renal unit, with a continuing overall mortality rate of about 40 per cent, and an increased demand for mobile dialysis with a sharp rise in the mortality of these patients.

In summary it can be seen that acute renal failure is a very complex disorder with a high mortality. It can arise from a vast number of causes and requires experienced judgement to assess the priorities of investigation and treatment of the various components of the illness. Great advantage has been gained by the introduction of peritoneal dialysis and by the simplification of haemodialysis by techniques used in chronic renal dialysis. Many cases are now prevented by the proper use of intravenous fluids and diuretics, but advances in general medical treatment are producing an increasing proportion of severely ill patients who may die of the original disease despite treatment of renal failure. This is the great challenge of the future.

QUESTIONNAIRE on Acute Renal Failure

Out of 35 questionnaires sent, 34 replies were received and of these 26 were suitable, and obtained in time, to be presented at the Symposium. Only 11 or the 26 units were functioning in 1962. The 26 units between them claimed to serve a population of 41 000 000. The patients treated by these units are shown in Table 9.8. The 433 renal transplants done compares accurately with the figure of 465 reported by the Department of Health and Social Security for the year ending 31 January 1973 (see Ref. 6) In fact, all the major transplant centres were included in the 26 units.

Table 9.8 Patients treated by 26 renal units

Home dialysis		568
Hospital dialysis		422
Renal transplant		433
Acute renal failure		590 (29%)
	Total	2013

Patients with acute renal failure numbered 590, some 29 per cent of the total of all patients treated (although no doubt some patients receiving transplants are also recorded as dialysis patients). The results of treatment related to the broad aetiological groups is given in Table 9.9.

The lowest mortality is among surgical patients with obstetric cases maintaining their enviable reputation with a mortality of 10 per cent. The author has long wondered whether the low mortality of obstetric cases is due to factors other than the natural history of the disease. The anxiety to prevent maternal mortality.

Table 9.9 Acute Renal Failure

Cause	Total	Died	Mortality
Medical	230	84	36%
Surgical	247	132	53%
Trauma	48	24	50%
Obstetric	39	4	10%
Other	26	12	46%
Total	590	256	43%

Table 9.10

	Where do you treat acute renal failure?	Where do you think acute renal failure should be treated?
Special acute unit	11	16
Intensive care ward	4	13
General medical ward	16	2
Chronic dialysis ward	2	0

almost always ensures that these patients are referred to renal units, and referred early.

Only nine units have done mobile dialysis and only four would be prepared to do so as policy.

The question relating to where acute renal failure is being treated and where units would prefer to treat produced the interesting replies set out in Table 9.10. Whereas the majority now treat in general medical wards their actual preference would be for special acute units or intensive care units. Several units gave multiple preferences so that the total view expressed exceed 26.

Questions 8 and 9 were framed to produce dogmatic answers concerning preference between peritoneal and haemodialysis because it is well known that views among different units have been polarised in the past. In reply six units refused to be drawn and stated that they used either technique as appropriate to the needs of the patients. Four units were definitely for haemo-

Table 9.11 Treatment of acute renal failure by choice (1)

First Choice	Units	Patients	Average/Unit
Haemodialsysis	4	115	28
Peritoneal dialysis	16	349	21
'Either'	6	126	21
Total	26	590	23

Table 9.12 Treatment of acute renal failure by choice (2)

First Choice	Units	Patients	Average
Peritoneal dialysis	2	166	83
Peritoneal dialysis	14	183	13
Haemodialysis	4	115	28
'Either'	6	126	21
Total	26	590	23

dialysis as the first choice and 16 units for peritoneal dialysis. The patients treated, and the average number per unit, is shown in Table 9.11. It seems to show an overall similarity of intake per year, with the 'haemodialysis' units in the lead. However, these figures were distorted by the large number (166) of patients treated by two units alone who declared for peritoneal dialysis. Separating these two units from the other 14 the results are presented in Table 9.12. From this it can be seen that there is a definite tendency for units with a preference for peritoneal dialysis to admit considerably less patients with acute renal failure than other units. The average was 13 per year, or approximately one per month. The anonymity of units was assurred, so that it must suffice to say that there exist special reasons for the extraordinary high intake of two units compared to the rest. However, it is very apparent that the selection of patients at each unit is very different. This is demonstrated in Table 9.13 which presents mortality by first choice of treatment. There is a difference of 50 and 18 per cent mortality rates which seems excessive unless

Table 9.13 Mortality by first choice of treatment

	Units	Patients	Mortality
Peritoneal dialysis	1	117	50%
Peritoneal dialysis	1	49	18%
Peritoneal dialysis	14	183	41%
Haemodialysis	4	115	50%
Either	6	126	50%
Total	26	590	43%

Table 9.14 Mortality by first choice of treatment and aetiology of acute renal failure

	Units	Medical	Surgical	Trauma
Either	6	32%	70%	43%
Haemodialysis	4	53%	53%	33%
Peritoneal dialysis	14	36%	48%	56%
Peritoneal dialysis	1	44%	54%	60%
Peritoneal dialysis	1	21%	12%	Nil (no patients)

different classes of patient are being treated.

To explore this further the mortality rates of medical, surgical and trauma cases, arranged according to first choice of treatment of all units is given in Table 9.14. Two striking points are apparent. Firstly, regardless of first choice of treatment, the mortality rates vary greatly in each category. Secondly, regardless of actual mortality rates, in units preferring haemodialysis or prepared to use it, the mortality rate for trauma is less than for surgical cases, while in all units preferring peritoneal dialysis the mortality rate for trauma is higher than in surgical cases.

Concerning the incidence of acute renal failure no unit thought it was increased, eight thought it to be decreasing, 16 static and only two modestly admitted that they did not know.

Twenty-one units claimed to encourage local hospitals to contact them when they had a case of acute renal failure, and five said frankly that they did not.

Asked for suggestions as to how the mortality of acute renal failure might be lowered by far the most common reply was for earlier referral of patients, a view with which the author is in complete agreement.

Comments

The purpose of the questionnaire, as stated, was to obtain information concerning the incidence and current attitudes to the treatment of acute renal failure. It was deliberately simple, and no pretence is made that the replies consistute hard facts capable of statistical analysis or dogmatic conclusions.

Probably the most reliable information concerns the number treated and the mortality rate. A total of 590 patients with acute renal failure were treated by the 26 units and 334 survived. In terms of useful life prolonged, therefore, it is quite possible that the efforts expended on treating these patients produced results comparable to those of renal transplantation. If so, it confirms our belief that acute renal failure is worthy of the highest possible priority in treatment. That this is a widely shared belief is confirmed by the majority of units wishing to treat patients in either special units or intensive care units. An interesting point concerning the incidence of acute renal failure is brought out by the questionnaire. As there were only 11 units operational in 1962 they would have had to treat an approximate average of 53 patients each to deal with 590 patients, and there is little doubt that none of them treated any such number in 1962. Furthermore, a large number of cases of acute renal failure are now treated in general hospitals or intensive care units, possibly it seems, up to twice the total treated in renal units. It follows, therefore, that whatever may be happening to the incidence of acute renal failure the number of patients being treated must definitely have increased.

References

1. Fry, I.K. and Cattell, W.R. (1971). Radiology in the diagnosis of acute renal failure. *Brit. Med. Bull.,* **27,** 148–152
2. Shaldon, S., Silva, H., Pmeroy, J., Rae, A.I. and Rosen, S.M. (1964). Percutaneous femoral venous catherization and reusable dialysers in the treatment of acute renal failure. *Proc. Amer. Soc. for Artificial Internal Organs.*
3. Kopp, K.F., Gutch, C.F. and Kolff, W.J. (1972). Single needle dialysis. *Proc. Amer. Soc. for Artificial Internal Organs*

4. Kennedy, A.C., Burton, J.A., Luke, R.G., Briggs, J.D., Lindsay, R.M., Allison, M.E.M., Edward, J. and Dargie, H.J. (19 ?). Factors affecting the prognosis in acute renal failure *Quart. J. Med.*, **42,** 165 73–86
5. Stott, R.B., Ogg, C.S., Cameron, J.S. and Bewick, M. (1972). Why the persistently high mortality in acute renal failure? *Lancet,* **2,** 75–78
6. *Health Trends,* **5,** (May 1973). Number 2. Department of Health and Social Security.

Discussion – Third Session

Dr Shaldon (National Kidney Centre, London)

This is a loaded question based on your suggestions. It seems that acute renal failure is passed it period of infancy and adolescence in terms of selection. I notice that Dr Lindsay was prepared to dialyse 80 year olds and was prepared to accept that 80 per cent were going to die. I would like to know what his age limit is for long term dialysis patients and whether he can rationalise the cost of acute dialysis in the old versus the cost of maintenance dialysis in the old.

Dr Lindsay (Glasgow)

It is rather a nasty question to answer. The way I think about it is that with acute renal failure, although there is such poor survival in the older people, you can never really spot a patient that you can say will not survive. I am sure we have all seen patients who have not really got much chance, who have in fact walked out and been quite well thereafter, so I think that in acute renal failure you must dialyse everybody. It is a potentially reversible situation, and if you have an acute unit with its own machines, not taking up space which is being used for chronic dialysis patients, I think that takes care of that. Our own feelings about chronic dialysis are that we have a rough upper age limit of 55.

Dr Mallick (Manchester)

I think we feel in Manchester very strongly on the points made by each speaker. Over the last year or so we have had available a good intensive care unit. Our results until then have always been very much in line with the results which were spoken about, but have improved over the last 18 months or so, and they show a survival rate now of about 70 per cent. One of the real difficulties we have in renal failure is that many of these patients die very early before we can get on to any combined therapy, and we feel that intensive care, (our unit is in fact part of an intensive care unit) with a number of physicians and surgeons who are interested in the problem together with the facilities and the nursing staff, can make a real dent in the mortality. I think we tend to make ourselves pessimistic because we get so many patients who are really too ill when they arrive for us to do much for, and , if we can get them over the first few days in the circumstances I described and I think Dr Flynn has put over very clearly, the mortality rate is nothing like as bad as the overall figures might suggest.

Dr Flynn (Halton) *The only thing I would say about that is that we also see seriously ill patients in intensive care units who we get to quite early. At this very moment our team is in Reading dialysing a patient, and the doctor in charge is here, Dr Price, and he can tell you that he in fact called us very early and we got there and dialysed him before the blood urea reached 250 mg. That was a week yesterday and we are still there and we are still dialysing and things are getting out of hand.* (Editor's privileged addendum – the patient eventually survived after 29 haemodialyses).

Peters *I think that you make the point that the kind of patients being treated are changing very much. In our hospital I am not sure, but I think the major single cause of acute renal failure is post by-pass surgery. Now even that particular practice in our own hospital has changed very much in recent years. Progressively one, two or three heart valves are being replaced almost routinely, and in this population of patients we see them very early and still find that they do badly, as you have indicated. We had one situation which was really quite interesting and quite instructive. We had a patient who had bacterial endocarditis who developed acute renal failure and that patient had his heart valve replaced while he was still oliguric. He had prolonged oliguria, and the whole thing went through very nicely, whereas among the other patients who develop acute renal failure post operatively are often those patients who are in fact systemically very sick to start off with, and often they have been on very large doses of drugs and diuretics etc. to control their heart failure. I think that this distinction is quite important.*

Lindsay *We can make a similar comment as well. There are two groups of surgical patients who fare very badly. As you say the by-pass patient and also the patient with severe burns who develop acute* *renal failure and our experience is that if they are ill enough to develop acute renal failure, they die. There is not really too much one can do about it in spite of dialysis.*

Dr McGeown (Belfast)

If I may make a comment to Dr Lindsay. I think your slide relating age to mortality is very misleading. You have shown an earlier slide in which for instance the best prognosis was the obstetrics ones. Now, your younger age group is bound to be loaded by that and some of the very severe surgical situations, for instance ruptured abdominal aneurysm, where the mortality is 100 per cent that will weight the older ones. I prefer to look on it as to the aetiological situation. I unhappily have a fair bit of experience of severe trauma due to gun shots and blast wounds. These are almost all in young adults, mostly male, although there is the odd female, and the prognosis is related to the severity of the injury. As Dr Flynn said multiple limb injuries are usually compatible with survival but those that are penetrated injuries of the abdomen particularly when there is multiple lacerations of the intestines with a lot of faecal staining almost all of them die and age can be eliminated. I do not mind if I see them with a ruptured liver with a pack in it or a bit of kidney blown away or the diaphragm ruptured or a chest injury but if they have multiple faecal staining as well as these other injuries and loss of limbs then they never survive. The limb ones may be different and they may be short of shunt sites but they nearly all do survive.

Lindsay

The only slight comment I would make on that is that if you break down our own group into just say the surgical patients there is still this relationship between age and mortality.

Shaldon

I would like to ask a question now regarding whether it is policy for intensive care units to have as part of its equipment an artificial kidney.

Dr Robson (Edinburgh)

Well I think that is a question that we would all perhaps have different ideas. It has certainly been my impression that in most of the renal units which run acute renal failure service on a sizeable scale they are in point of fact equipped as intensive care units, sometimes adjacent to it, sometimes separated, but they are nevertheless equipped for ECGs, central venous pressure, var-

ious cardiac monitoring, assisted respiration etc. and I do not know the extent to which this conflict that Dr Mallick raised between intesive care units and non-

Shaldon *You misread my question James. We have heard that Halton are going to an intensive care unit in Reading to do a dialysis. My question is why?*

Flynn *Who else will go?*

Shaldon *So it is not therefore Health Service Policy to have an artificial kidney machine in every intensive care unit?*

Flynn *As far as I am aware it is not. I mean the reason why as a Service unit we are going now to Reading is partly because we wish to keep the expertise of mobile dialysis practised for our own purposes when we need it, which is rarely.*

Robson *Perhaps the point which Stanley is making, and if it isn't clear I am sure he will excuse me, but I think it is an important one which comes to my mind. There is a policy about maintenance chronic dialysis and there is a national policy about transplantation whatever you may think of it. It does not seem to me there ever was a policy about acute renal failure. It grew up in a very haphazard way. Now you say there were 35 units and your population covered was 41 million.*

Flynn *Not quite. 26 units covered 41 million population.*

Robson *And the average number of patients I think per year was something between 20 and 30. Now we do not know the distribution of these units geographically, although a cover of 41 million is obviously a large proportion of the population, but we do not know whether there are lakes of untreated or badly treated acute renal failure. Dr Brun said this morning that he thought that we should never forget acute renal failure. One of the astonishing things that I've found going around the world is that you go into very large hospitals and they say they have never heard of acute renal failure, they do not see it, and I am sure that may well be the experience of others.*

Dr Goodwin (London)

I should like to comment on Dr Flynn's data on the incidence of acute renal failure. Of course the figures that he gives reflect the incidence as seen by us who work in renal units and not those seen throughout the whole country. I should like to comment on some work that Dr David Fisher at the London has been doing in the North-East Metropolitan region which has a population of something like 3¼ million. He has been scouring almost every hospital to try and establish exactly how many patients have acute renal failure in this region and the results are rather surprising. If I could just comment on one year's figures for acute renal failure following surgery – 12 cases either arose in renal centres or were referred to renal centres and over twice that figure, 29, developed renal failure in perpheral hospitals. So that for every case of renal failure we see in renal units there are probably two outside we never see. Now there is even rather more sinister development on this. That is, that of those 29 in outside hospitals, of the 23 which died only four had received peritoneal dialysis, none had received haemodialysis and of the six survivors only three had received peritoneal dialysis. Whereas of the 12 cases treated in renal centres, seven died and only one case did not receive either peritoneal dialysis or haemodialysis. So it looks as though there are a great many cases dying outside renal units which are not being treated adequately or even given a change of treatment.

Robson

Thank you very much. 'I think that is a very interesting observation.

Flynn

I am delighted to hear that this study was done. This was what I was suggesting, that we need to know a great deal more. I said that there was 590 patients treated in renal units and I did not want to guess, but I was assuming there were probably twice that number occurring outside.

Dr Prosser (Southampton)

I am an anaesthetist. I would be interested to hear as to whether there is such a thing as incipient renal failure or not. I tend to think with the Glasgow people that there is and I would agree with them. There certainly is in the theatre. You see patients who are going to get renal failure almost certainly unless something is done about it pretty quickly. Now it is quite obvious you have got to replace blood volume and all the rest of it. I would like to endorse what I think Dr Lindsay said that we believe and teach there is a place for either mannitol, ethacrynic acid or frusemide in this situation, and I would like to ask the brains that are here which of these three agents is the best, and whether they believe that Starr's work on the improvement in glomerular filtration as a result of ethacrynic acid could lead them to say that perhaps this is the best choice or would they not use it at all.

Robson *Dr Lindsay would obviously use it.*

Lindsay *I would like to say thank you very much. It is nice to have some friends. It is difficult. I do not have any data to suggest which is the better, or how to do it in fact. I think we all agree that although we all have the impression, to actually prove that it did work would involve a very major double blind trial which would be impossible with the heterogenecity of the type of patients, so it is really very difficult certainly for me to say which I think is best. Our impression is that mannitol is best and we are not really too impressed with frusemide. Frankly in fact we give mannitol and if this does not work we give a jumbo dose of frusemide intravenously and in some it does seem to work.*

Flynn *I would like to add to that. It seems to me that if you use mannitol in high risk circumstances there is evidence which suggests, but does not prove, that the incidence of acute renal failure falls. I have not been personally quite so impressed with its use in more established acute renal failure, and I am worried about it is it does not work because, it is quite a dangerous stuff to be circulating, and I would have thought that under these circumstances frusemide is probably a safer drug.*

Joekes *I would entirely agree with those that think that mannitol works. I think we have clear evidence that it does at times. I am not convinced about Lasix. We have in a sense got some evidence about ethacrynic acid in patients who have failed to respond to mannitol, failed to respond to Lasix, who have then responded to to 50 mg of ethacrynic acid intravenously. These are entirely one single group of patients, namely those with major myocardial damage. These are the only ones we have ever seen who have* *responded like this, I think there are about five, quite dramatically, and have reversed the lesion, whatever it is, and have gone on to have non-oliguric failure. The one other thing that came in from work published by Ghosh and myself some years ago on Rheomacrodex. We studied eight patients in St. Thomas' Hospital who had open heart surgery and one of these having had priming with Rheomacrodex went into renal failure and we demonstrated in this group that Rheomacrodex is an excellent anti-diuretic agent, which is probably not ideal.*

Kerr *I do not think anyone is in doubt that there is such a condition as pre- renal uraemia which is corrected by adequate fluid replacement. What some of us are in doubt about is whether there is also a condition following fluid retention in which you can reverse the sequence of events by giving mannitol or frusemide. There is a well known delay of some hours sometimes before diuresis picks up after you have replaced the fluid and what we wondered is whether you merely squeeze a little urine out an hour or two before it would have come naturally.*

Robson *I would only make the point that it never seems to me surprising that the acute renal failure kidney in which not all the nephrons are clearly or totally ablated, that those which are surviving and operating are bound to respond in the normal pharmacological way both with mannitol and frusemide by increasing the urine flow. I have never been convinced that it increased urea or nitrogen excretion or, as you say, it would not have happened anyway.*

Peters *If we really want to have I believe it is, I believe it is not kind of argument or discussion, let me add my voice to the people of Glasgow to say that in our experience, which I am sure is as uncontrolled as Dr Kerr's (I wonder if he regularly gives frusemide or not?) is that in some patients in whom all the evidence suggests that, after proper fluid replacement, that they are going to get a acute renal failure that in some patients the administration of frusemide in large doses converts oliguric renal failure into non-oliguric renal failure. Now I do not know how it is in other places but it seems to me to be quite a useful state of affairs so far as the patient is concerned. So if that is the only claim to be made for frusemide in my view that justifies its use. What I am very disturb-*

ed by though, and I have recently travelled around the world fairly extensively, is going to various renal units to find a diversity of opinion. For example, one person, an ex-Glaswegian, Dr Linton, who I visited in London, Ontario, stated that in his view frusemide in these doses was practically nephrotoxic and it was folly to use it. Criminal negligence!

Brown *I wonder if we could have a few facts now instead of I believe, I have seen and maybe there and everywhere. We have studied 49 patients over the last five years. We analysed our data on mortality, just looking at post surgical acute renal failure, because I am sure that we really have to define all our groups very carefully and even amongst the post surgical acute renal failure we probably want to subdivide further, but it is always difficult to get enough patients to make analysis significant. We have seen 73 patients with post surgical acute renal failure, and most of them are post by-pass, the majority being post by-pass in abdominal surgery and in those we have given between 250 mg and 1 g of Lasix in 49 patients. Out of those 49 patients with the criteria of acute renal failure being a urinary sodium of above 10 mEq/litre, a UP urea ratio of 10:1 or less, and a UP osmolality ratio of 1:1 or less, (because I think we have to make these definitions very strict when we talk about our results); in those 49, four patients responded to frusemide in a way that obviated dialysis. Of seven others, four had a diuresis of more than 1.5 litres/day which was very useful in terms of nutrition, there were three, who had at first a diuresis and then subsequently became oliguric. These are facts as opposed to impressions.*

Appendix 1

QUESTIONNAIRE ON ACUTE RENAL FAILURE

1. WHEN DID UNIT OPEN? ....

2. POPULATION SERVED ....

3. NUMBER OF PATIENTS (RDT)
   (a) ON HOME DIALYSIS ....
   (b) ON HOSPITAL DIALYSIS ....

4. DOES YOUR UNIT DO RENAL TRANSPLANTS YES/NO

   IF YES, HOW MANY IN 1972 ......

   IF NO, HOW MANY OF YOUR PATIENTS WERE TRANSPLANTED ELSEWHERE IN 1972 ......

5. DO YOU TREAT ACUTE RENAL FAILURE YES/NO

   IF YES, HOW MANY IN 1972 ......

   CAN YOU COMPLETE THE FOLLOWING YES/NO

   CAUSES, NUMBERS, AND SURVIVAL OF ACUTE RENAL FAILURE PATIENTS TREATED IN 1972

CAUSE	NUMBER	LIVED	DIED
MEDICAL			
SURGICAL			
TRAUMA			
OBSTETRIC			
....			
....			
....			

6. DO YOU TREAT ACUTE RENAL FAILURE (Delete as appropriate)

    (a) IN CHRONIC DIALYSIS WARDS

    (b) IN A SPECIAL ACUTE UNIT

    (c) IN GENERAL MEDICAL WARDS

7. HAVE YOU EVER SENT AN ARTIFICIAL KIDNEY AND TEAM TO ANOTHER HOSPITAL YES/NO

    IF YES, IS THIS A REGULAR POLICY OF YOUR UNIT YES/NO

8. DO YOU USE PERITONEAL DIALYSIS (Delete as appropriate) IN ACUTE RENAL FAILURE

    (a) AS FIRST CHOICE IN ALL CASES

    (b) ONLY WHEN HAEMODIALYSIS IS UNSUITABLE

    (c) RARELY

9. DO YOU USE HAEMODIALYSIS (Delete as appropriate) IN ACUTE RENAL FAILURE

    (a) AS FIRST CHOICE IN ALL CASES

    (b) ONLY WHEN PERITONEAL DIALYSIS IS UNSUITABLE

    (c) RARELY

10. DO YOU THINK THE INCIDENCE OF ACUTE RENAL FAILURE IS

    (a) INCREASING

    (b) DECREASING (Delete as appropriate)

    (c) STATIC

11. WHERE DO YOU THINK ACUTE RENAL FAILURE SHOULD BE TREATED

    (a) IN SPECIAL RENAL CENTRES

    (b) IN GENERAL HOSPITALS (Delete as appropriate)

    (c) IN INTENSIVE CARE UNITS

12. DO YOU ENCOURAGE HOSPITALS IN YOUR AREA TO CONTACT YOU WHEN THERE IS A CASE OF ACUTE RENAL FAILURE

YES/NO

13. THE OVERALL MORTALITY RATE IN ACUTE RENAL FAILURE SEEMS TO BE ABOUT 50%. HAVE YOU ANY SUGGESTIONS AS TO HOW THIS MAY BE DECREASED?

Appendix 2

LIST OF PARTICIPANTS

Dr P. Ackrill	The London Hospital, Whitechapel
Dr R. Allison	East Birmingham Hospital
Dr J. Anderton	Western General, Edinburgh
Major M. Attia	Royal Army Medical College, Millbank
Dr R. Baillod	Royal Free Hospital, London
Mr A. Barnes	Queen Elizabeth Hospital, Birmingham
Dr R. Bibby	Royal Infirmary, Manchester
Dr Bisson	Royal Devon & Exeter Hospital, Exeter
Dr J. Blainey	Queen Elizabeth Hospital, Birmingham
Dr Bolton Jones	
Dr D. Boyle	Douglas, Isle of Man
Dr J. Briggs	Western Infirmary, Glasgow
Wg Cdr A. Broughton	I.P.T.M. RAF Halton
Dr C. Brown	Guy's Hospital, London
Captain G. Brown	Queen Alexandra Military Hospital, Millbank
Dr C. Brun	Copenhagen, Denmark
Dr M. Carmody	Jervis Street Hospital, Dublin
Lt Col. T. Carson	Tidworth Military Hospital
Dr Campbell MacKenzie	Southmead Hospital, Bristol
Dr W. Cattell	St. Bartholomew's Hospital, London
Miss M. Christian	Wexham Park Hospital, Slough
Sqn Ldr J. Christie	I.P.T.M., RAF Halton
Dr Clarke	
Surg. Lt P. Clarke	RNH Haslar
Dr A. Coakley	Royal Infirmary, Hull
Gp Capt. J.N.C. Cooke	PMRAF Hospital, Halton
Flt Lt R. Cooper	PMRAF Hospital, Halton
Lt Col. J. Cormack	Queen Alexandra Military Hospital, Millbank
Dr R. Crockett	The London Hospital, Whitechapel
Sqn Ldr S. Cullen	I.P.T.M., RAF Halton
Dr J. Curtis	Charing Cross Hospital, London
Dr Dargie	Royal Infirmary, Glasgow
Dr R Dathan	Royal South Hants Hospital, Portsmouth
Dr A. Davies	Royal Alexandra Hospital, Rhyl
Mr P. Dawson-Edwards	Queen Elizabeth Hospital, Birmingham

Dr W. Deutz	Royal Infirmary, Glasgow
Dr M. Doyle	Stoke Mandeville Hospital, Aylesbury
Dr D. Dukes	Coventry & Warwickshire Hospital, Coventry
Dr H. Dukes	Coventry & Warwickshire Hospital, Coventry
Dr M. Dunnill	Radcliffe Infirmary, Oxford
Dr W. Elliott	Royal Infirmary, Newcastle
Dr J. Eastwood	Charing Cross Hospital, London
Dr J. England	Sefton General Hospital, Liverpool
Dr D. Evans	Addenbrooke's Hospital, Cambridge
Flt Lt P. Fenwick	Medical Centre, RAF West Drayton
Major J. Findlow	Cambridge Military Hospital, Aldershot
Sqn Ldr W.R. Fitzgerald	Papworth Hospital, Cambridge
Wg Cdr C.T. Flynn	PMRAF Hospital, Halton
Wg Cdr D. Foster	Medical Centre, RAF Halton
Dr A. Frank	The London Hospital, Whitechapel
Mr J. Garland	North Manchester & Salford Hospitals
Dr M. Goggin	Kent & Canterbury Hospital, Canterbury
Dr F. Goldby	Royal Infirmary, Cardiff
Dr F. Goodwin	The London Hospital, Whitechapel
Dr P. Gower	Charing Cross Hospital, London
Dr C. Hall	Queen Elizabeth Hospital, Birmingham
Dr W. Halley	High Wycombe General Hospital, High Wycombe
Sqn Ldr R. Harris	PARAF Hospital, Wroughton, Swindon
Flt Lt D. Hawkes	Wolverhampton
Dr J. Hawkins	East Birmingham Hospital
Dr B. Hickson	St Bartholomews Hospital, London
Sqn Ldr A. Higginson	I.P.T.M., RAF Halton
Cp Capt. J. Hill	RAF Hospital, Ely, Cambs
Dr D. Hilton	Wordsley Hospital, Stourbridge
Dr A. Holmes	Royal Infirmary, Manchester
Surg. Lt N. Hopkin	Royal Naval Hospital, Haslar
Flt Lt J. Hopkirk	Wolverhampton
Dr P Horsey	Southampton General Hospital
Wg Cdr D. Hull	RAF Hospital, Gosford, Wolverhampton
Dr B. Hulme	St. Mary's Hospital, London
Gp Capt. F.D. Hutter	PMRAF Hospital, Halton
Mr R. Jackaman	Royal Postgraduate Medical School, Hammersmith
AVM Sir Ralph Jackson	RAF Central Medical Establishment, London
Dr A. Joekes	St. Philip's Hospital, London
Lt Col. W. Johnston	Queen Alexandra Military Hospital, Millbank
Wg Cdr F. Jones	I.P.T.M., RAF Halton

Dr N.F. Jones	St. Thomas' Hospital, London.
Surg. Lt P. Jones	Royal Naval Hospital, Haslar
Sqn Ldr P. Jowitt	PMRAF Hospital, Halton
Air Cdre H.B. Kelly	RAF Hospital, Wegberg, Germany
Dr D. Kenward	North Ormesby, Teeside
Professor D. Kerr	Royal Infirmary, Newcastle
Air Cdre A. Klidjian	PARAF Hospital, Wroughton, Swindon
Dr G. Ku	Royal Free Hospital, London
Dr A. Kulatilake	Royal Postgraduate Medical School, Hammersmith
Wg Cdr W. Larkworthy	RAF Hospital, Nocton Hall, Lincs.
Dr J. Lavender	Royal Postgraduate Medical School, Hammersmith
Dr S. Lavender	Royal South Hants Hospital, Portsmouth
Dr R. Lindsay	Royal Infirmary, Glasgow
Lt Col. I. Lister	Queen Alexandra Military Hospital, Millbank
Dr W. Loughridge	Westminster Hospital, London
Dr A. MacDougall	Stobhill Hospital, Glasgow
Major General R. MacFarlane	MOD, Lansdowne House
Dr J. MacGregor	Charing Cross Hospital, London
Dr C. MacKintosh	Westminster Hospital, London
Mr J. Maddocks	Royal Infirmary, Cardiff
Dr N. Mallick	Royal Infirmary Manchester
Air Cdre J. Malcolm	RAF Central Medical Establishment, London
Dr D. Malone	City Hospital, Nottingham
Dr F. Marsh	The London Hospital, Whitechapel
Dr A. Martin	Royal Infirmary, Sunderland
Gp Capt. T. Mason	I.P.T.M., RAF Halton
Wg Cdr McCafferty	RAF Hospital, Nocton Hall, Lincs.
Dr M. McGeown	Belfast City Hospital, Belfast
Gp Capt. I. McIntosh	I.H.M.T., RAF Halton
Surg. Lt M. McLeod	Royal Naval Hospital, Haslar
Flt Lt M. Melvin	RAF Hospital, Nocton Hall, Lincs
Dr R. Middleton	Royal Alexandra Hospital, Rhyl
Dr P. Millard	Radcliffe Infirmary, Oxford
Flt Lt Mills	
Mr J. Moorhead	Royal Free Hospital, London
Air Cdre R. Mortimer	I.P.T.M., RAF Halton
Mr C. Newman	Queen Elizabeth Hospital, Birmingham
Sqn Ldr Newrick	I.P.T.M., RAF Halton
Professor W. O'Dwyer	Jervis Street Hospital, Dublin
Major Oldrey	Royal Hospital, Woolwich
Dr E. Paice	Stoke Manderville Hospital, Alyesbury
Dr A Parker	Southmead Hospital, Bristol
Colonel Parker	Military Hospital, Colchester

Lt Col. E. Parry	Cambridge Military Hospital, Aldershot
Dr K. Peters	Hammersmith Hospital
Dr P. Philalithis	St. Philip's Hospital, London
Dr M. Phillips	Charing Cross Hospital, London
Dr M. Platts	Royal Hospital, Sheffield
Dr D.G. Price	Royal Berks Hospital, Reading
Surg. Lt A. Procter	Royal Naval Hospital, Haslar
Dr D. Prosser	Westminster Hospital, London
Dr J.S. Pryer	Norfolk & Norwich Hospital, Norwich
Flt Lt D.J. Rainford	PMRAF Hospital, Halton
Dr A. Ralston	Withington Hospital, Manchester
Flt Lt P.C.V. Ramage	PMRAF Hospital, Halton
Surg. Lt L. Ramsay	Royal Naval Hospital, Haslar
Dr P. Read	Hoechst Pharmaceuticals
Dr A. Rees	Guy's Hospital, London
Surg. Lt B. Reid	Royal Naval Hospital, Haslar
Dr G. Relwani	Royal Infirmary, Cardiff
Dr B. Robinson	East Birmingham Hospital, Birmingham
Dr D. Robson	St Philip's Hospital, London
Dr J.S. Robson	Royal Infirmary, Edingburgh
Dr P. Row	Guy's Hospital, London
Dr L. Sevitt	Hillingdon Hospital, Middx
Professor R. Shackman	Royal Postgraduate Medical School, Hammersmith Hospital
Dr S. Shaldon	National Kidney Centre, London
Flt Lt Sharwood-Smith	PMRAF Hospital, Halton
Dr T. Sherwood	Institute of Urology, London
A.V.M. Sir Ernest Sidey,	MOD Tavistock Square, London
Dr T. Silver	Stoke Manderville Hospital, Aylesbury
Wg Cdr C.E. Simpson	PMRAF Hospital, Halton
Dr Sinclair	
Mr A. Siviter	Queen Elizabeth Hospital, Birmingham
Sqn Ldr J. Smith	RAF Hospital, Nocton Hall, Lincs
Dr S. Smith	Coventry & Warwickshire Hospital, Coventry
Air Cdre. C.J. Soutar	PMRAF Hospital, Halton
Gp Capt. M. Sparks	Medical Survey Office, Gloucester
Lt Col. J. Stewart	Royal Army Medical College, Millbank
Dr P. Sullivan	Coventry & Warwickshire Hospital, Coventry
Gp Capt P.D. Sutton	PMRAF Hospital, Halton
Dr A. Sweatman	Royal Free Hospital, London
Dr A. Syed	Hillingdon Hospital, Middx
Dr P. Tasker	Charing Cross Hospital, London
Dr I Thangkhiew	Wolverhampton
Dr Thill	
Dr W.B. Thomson	High Wycombe General Hospital

Sqn Ldr A. Tredre	PARAF Hospital, Wroughton, Swindon
Dr H. Tunstall-Pedoe	The London Hospital, Whitechapel
Wg Cdr K. Underwood-Ground	I.P.T.M., RAF Halton
Mr Z. Varghese	Royal Free Hospital, London
Capt C. Volkers	Queen Alexandra Military Hospital, Millbank
Professor H. de Wardener	Charing Cross Hospital, London
Surg. Lt M. White	Royal Naval Hospital, Haslar
Surg. Lt Williams	Royal Naval Hospital, Plymouth
Dr Winchester	Royal Infirmary, Glasgow
Dr A. Wing	St. Thomas' Hospital, London
Dr W. Winney	Royal Infirmary, Edinburgh
Dr R. Woods	Whipps Cross Hospital, Leytonstone, London
Dr R. Wordingham	Central Ammunition Centre, Basingstoke
Dr F. Wright	Royal Alexandra Hospital, Rhyl
Dr K. Youseff	Royal Free Hospital, London
Flt Lt Winstur	RAF Hospital, Cosford, Wolverhampton

INDEX

GPSR Compliance

The European Union's (EU) General Product Safety Regulation (GPSR) is a set of rules that requires consumer products to be safe and our obligations to ensure this.

If you have any concerns about our products, you can contact us on ProductSafety@springernature.com

In case Publisher is established outside the EU, the EU authorized representative is:

Springer Nature Customer Service Center GmbH
Europaplatz 3
69115 Heidelberg, Germany

Batch number: 10584444

Printed by Printforce, the Netherlands